Stepping into Palliative Care 2

Care and practice

Second Edition

Edited by

Jo Cooper
Macmillan Clinical Nurse Specialist in Palliative Care

Foreword by
Philip Burnard
Professor of Nursing and Vice Dean for Academic Affairs
School of Nursing and Midwifery Studies
Wales College of Medicine
Cardiff University

Radcliffe Publishing
Oxford • Seattle

Radcliffe Publishing Ltd
18 Marcham Road
Abingdon
Oxon OX14 1AA
United Kingdom

www.radcliffe-oxford.com
Electronic catalogue and worldwide online ordering facility.

British Library Cataloguing in Publication Data

A catalogue record for this book is available from the British Library.

ISBN-10: 1 85775 792 0
ISBN-13: 978 1 85775 792 7

Typeset by Advance Typesetting Ltd, Oxford
Printed and bound by TJ International Ltd, Padstow, Cornwall

Contents

Foreword

It is good to see this excellent book appearing in a second edition. The text has been thoroughly updated but, as with the previous edition, the focus remains practical.

Considerable thought has gone into the production of this book. The layout is clear and makes for easy reading. The chapters are written by subject experts who are also excellent communicators. In this field, the issue of communication is a vital one and it is good to see that those who practise in it can also convey their ideas clearly and practically.

That the book appears in a second edition indicates how helpful it has been to its 'first generation' of readers. I can imagine many people benefiting from this book: students on diploma and degree programmes, clinical practitioners and a range of other carers. It will also be useful to nurses in other fields who need or want to gather an understanding of what palliative care is about. It will also be a valuable resource in the library of any hospice or palliative care organisation. I found the book both educational and enlightening.

Nursing, in all fields, is turning to evidence-based practice: to attempting to identify 'what works' and 'what works best'. Usually this approach involves drawing on a range of research projects to identify best practice. However, despite researchers' best efforts, there is still a need to draw upon practitioners' experience – particularly in such a 'sensitive' area as palliative care. I am delighted to be associated with the wealth of information that is to be found in this book. I congratulate both the editor and the contributors for all their work and know that the book will help both patients and nursing staff, in very many ways.

Philip Burnard
August 2006

Philip Burnard PhD, RN
Professor of Nursing and Vice Dean for Academic Affairs
School of Nursing and Midwifery Studies
Wales College of Medicine
Cardiff University

Setting the scene

The first edition of *Stepping into Palliative Care* was primarily intended for those new to the field of palliative care. The second edition is aimed at a broader readership, crossing all role boundaries and differing levels of expertise. Within *Stepping into Palliative Care 1: relationships and responses* and *Stepping into Palliative Care 2: care and practice* there are many new chapters not only addressing the practical, technical and fundamental care issues but looking deeper and wider into *how* being a person with cancer, and the family, feels. Issues of existentialism, the human experience of *being*, and the nature of therapeutic relating, have been comprehensively embraced. *Stepping into Palliative Care 1 and 2* can be applied to practice by the novice and experienced practitioner, and aim to present illustrations of best theory and practice.

As palliative care travels its own unique and distinctive voyage, the significance of attending to the spiritual, social, emotional and psychological needs of the patient and family are paramount in the provision of care. This second edition looks at not only the need for empirical knowledge, but also the aesthetic knowledge, and art of caring. It aims to capture the essence of what it *means* to be *alongside* suffering: care that goes beyond words, capturing souls, spirit and compassion.

It is essential to remember the *true* meaning of palliative care in a time where we are politically conscious of the need to demonstrate clinical effectiveness and to determine outcomes of care. Two opposing paradigms, on one continuum: *both* can be met and intertwined.

In order to meet the requirements of the individual who is exposed to palliative care, the professional needs education and training targeted at the *how to* element of professional practice and patient management. For the professional who is in daily or occasional contact with the patient, family and significant others affected by cancer, it is an integral part of his or her professional daily life. For the professional to be able to identify problems and monitor treatment, interventions and support services, it is essential there is a clear pathway of perception of the active role that each one of us plays, and participates in – be that before, during and/or after palliative care has been accessed.

In *Stepping into Palliative Care 1 and 2*, each chapter builds on the last to offer an overview of the needs relating to the individual who encounters palliative care. Where applicable, a chapter makes full and effective use of *at-a-glance* features including boxes, tables, figures, self-assessment, reflection and case scenarios. The *'To learn more'* sections point the reader in the direction of further knowledge and information. At the end of the book there is a *'Useful contacts'* section that can provide more information, advice and guidance for the professional, patient, family and significant others.

This edition can be used as a starting point to further education and training. It attempts to provide some sensitive answers, discuss some issues surrounding palliative care, and direct the reader towards further development.

If you lose hope, somehow you lose the vitality that keeps life moving, you lose that courage to be, that quality that helps you go on in spite of it all. And so today I still have a dream. (*The Trumpet of Conscience*, Martin Luther King, Jr)

Jo Cooper
August 2006

Cautionary note

Throughout this book, reference is made to drugs and dosage. The authors and editor have made every effort to check the accuracy of this information and to ensure that information is up-to-date. However, it should be noted that drugs, dosage and indications can change as current research and developments provide new supporting evidence. It is essential that the prescribing individual check the drug, dosage and indications, at the time of the proposed prescribing, with current recommendations. Moreover, the individual administering the medication should check the evidence available at that time. The pharmacist is a valuable resource for all aspects of drug administration and prescribing information. The editor would recommend cross-referencing from the latest edition of Twycross R, Wilcock A, Charlesworth S *et al. Palliative Care Formulary* (Radcliffe Publishing).

List of contributors

Editor

Jo Cooper BSc (Hons) (Palliative Nursing), Dip Oncology, RGN, Specialist Practitioner – adult nursing (palliative care)
Macmillan Clinical Nurse Specialist in Palliative Care
Winkleigh, Devon

Contributors

Lynn Basford MA, BA (Hons), RN, NDN, Cert CPT, RNT, Cert Ed
Dean and Professor of Health Sciences
University of Lethbridge
Alberta, Canada

Mary Brooks RGN, RCM, Dip in Palliative Care
Clinical Nurse Specialist
North Devon Hospice
Barnstaple, North Devon

Mark Collier BA (Hons), RN, ONC, RCNT, RNT, V300
Nurse Consultant – Tissue Viability
Pilgrim Hospital
Practitioner/Health Lecturer
University of Nottingham

Jo Cooper
Winkleigh, Devon

Andrew Dickman MSc, MRPharmS
Specialist Principal Pharmacist
Palliative Care Team
Whiston Hospital
Merseyside

Jenny Forrest MBCHB, MRCP, MRCGP
Specialist Registrar Clinic Oncology
Royal Devon and Exeter Hospital
Exeter, Devon

Mezzi Franklin RN, RM, DN, MA Dramatherapy, B Phil Complementary Health Studies, ITEC Massage, ITEC Aromatherapy, Cert Ed
Clinical Nurse Specialist
North Devon District Hospital
Barnstaple, North Devon

James Gilbert FRCP, ILTM
Medical Director
Exeter Hospiscare
Exeter, Devon

Julie Hewett RGN, Dip N, BSc (Hons)
Macmillan Head and Neck Clinical Nurse Specialist
Torbay Hospital
Torquay, Devon

Susanna Hill MBChB, DCH, MRCGP, Dip Pall Med
General Practitioner
Macmillan General Practitioner Facilitator
Caen Medical Centre
Braunton, North Devon

Annie Hogg RGN, Dip NS
Clinical Nurse Specialist
North Devon Hospice
Barnstaple, North Devon

Trevor Mitten BSc (Hons), Dip Nurs, RGN, Orthopaedic Nursing Cert, FETC
Clinical Nurse Specialist in Palliative Care
North Devon Hospice
Barnstaple, North Devon

Mark Napier MBBS, FRCP
Consultant Medical Oncologist
Royal Devon and Exeter Hospital, Exeter
North Devon District Hospital
Barnstaple, North Devon

David Oliver BSc, FRCGP
Consultant in Palliative Medicine
Wisdom Hospice, Rochester
Honorary Senior Lecturer in Palliative Care
Kent Institute of Medicine and Health Sciences
University of Kent

Jenny Penson MA, SRN, HV, Cert Ed, RNT, Cert Counselling
Teacher, Therapist and Writer
Barnstaple, North Devon

Mandy Redgrove BA (Hons), PGCE, CQSW, MA, Dip Counselling
Emotional and Spiritual Care Services Manager
North Devon Hospice
Barnstaple, North Devon

Audrey Smyth NNEB
Volunteer in bereavement team
North Devon Hospice
Barnstaple, North Devon
Nursery officer in therapeutic family child protection team (retired)

Reverend Professor Stephen G Wright FRCN, MBE
Faculty of Health and Social Care
St Martin's College, Lancaster
Editor, *Spirituality and Health International*
Chairman, The Sacred Space Foundation
Mungrisedale, Cumbria

Acknowledgements

To each author for their rigorous hard work, dedication, passion and commitment in producing quality text for *Stepping into Palliative Care 1 and 2* despite continuous heavy workloads. For completing chapters willingly, sharing knowledge, expertise, personal knowledge and experience and adding to the richness of this second edition – thank you.

Thank you to Gillian Nineham for having faith in me, and to Lisa Abbott, Jamie Etherington, Paula Peebles and the team at Radcliffe Publishing.

To the chapter reviewers for their expertise and constructive comments: Susanna Hill, Louise Whitehead, Sue Lloyd, Claire Taylor, Sheena McCullough and Philip D Cooper – thank you.

To my immediate team colleagues who have provided a source of strength, inspiration, vision, wisdom and encouragement – thank you.

To David, my advisor, administrator, greatest critic and my best friend, without whom what follows would never have been.

Any errors and omissions are the sole responsibility of the editor.

Jo Cooper
August 2006

Dedication

Where my journey into palliative care began ...
... to the nurses and medical staff of the bedded unit, St Nicholas Hospice, Bury St Edmunds, West Suffolk.
... and to where the journey continues ...
... to the nurses and medical staff of the bedded unit, North Devon Hospice, Barnstaple, Devon ...
... special people, who touch our lives in a certain way, and having known them, we will never be the same. **Thank you.**

To our third generation – our hope for the future ...

We should not let our fears hold us back from pursuing our hopes.
(John F Kennedy)

Jo Cooper
August 2006

Chapter 1

Assessment in palliative care

Mary Brooks

Pre-reading exercise 1.1
Time: 10 minutes

Consider in what ways an assessment process can be helpful to:

- you
- other team members
- the patient.

What is assessment?

Assessment is a continuous, ongoing process, beginning even before the professional and patient identify problematic issues. Once the provisional care plan has been agreed, assessment continues throughout to ensure interventions and treatment are adjusted to meet the patient's and family's needs. However, there is usually a point when the professional, patient and family sit down and systematically draw together information required to decide on the exact nature of the problem and how best to move forward.[1] The primary aim of assessment is three-fold:

1 *Information* – gather accurate information (*listening to their story*) about the:
   - person
   - family
   - illness
   - associated problems.
2 *Identify* – factors associated with the illness.
3 *Coping strategies* – explore strengths and weaknesses and the person's ability to cope with, and play a pivotal role in the management of, the illness and identified problems.[1]

To be effective, assessment involves two-way communications,[2] enabling patient and family to express

- hopes
- fears
- expectations

and to receive information about the illness, interventions and treatment. This requires sensitivity and skill, which develops with experience and knowledge.

Why is assessment important?

Symptoms related to cancer do not take place in isolation. Cancer causes other problems. Therefore, throughout assessment the professional must consider the holistic needs of the patient and family covering the following aspects of the individual's life:

- physical
- psychological
- social
- emotional
- economical
- spiritual.[3]

While including highly clinical aspects, the professionals' role is primarily to facilitate self-help. It is acknowledged that the patient is the expert in his or her own care and needs[4] and the professionals' role is to facilitate that expertise, to identify problems, and offer appropriate interventions and treatment, to achieve the individual's chosen goal. Consequently, in order to plan care it is necessary to have good information about the patient's and family's:

- inclinations
- strengths
- abilities
- problems
- difficulties.

Other agencies, professional and lay, may be involved with the patient and family. Therefore, it is essential to identify each, and the role each plays in the individual's life. This avoids overlap, enhances coordination and effective interdisciplinary work and directs resources to the direct care of the individual.

The assessment questions are three-fold:

1 What can I do for the patient and family?
2 What can the patient and family do?
3 How can I help the patient and family maintain their independence?[1]

What should assessment include?

Every individual has a story to tell. Encourage the patient and family member to tell his or her story:

- using their words
- in their own time.

This may be time consuming but it is time well spent. Without a holistic picture, intervention and treatment is ineffective. Only when you have decided what information is needed can you clarify:

- why you need it
- what you will do with it.

During assessment ask yourself:

- what decisions do the patient, family and I have to make?
- what information is needed to aid the decision-making process?[1]

The process of assessment

Assessment should take place in a safe, confidential environment, with sensitivity towards issues of race, culture, gender, sexuality, religion and age. The way the assessment is conducted and information is collected, influences the rapport between the professional, patient and family, which in turn will affect the process of any interventions that follow.[1] Patients most likely to engage are those who feel the professional is warm, accepting, understanding, knowledgeable and genuinely wants to work with them.[1]

Assessment provides an opportunity to gain insight into the illness and its impact on the individual's and family's life. If assessment is thorough and part of mutual openness and understanding, effective treatment and intervention can be made jointly on the basis of a shared understanding.

Assessment tools

While helpful in aiding diagnosis or symptom severity, assessment tools do not take the place of a willingness to listen and the ability to understand the patient and family. Assessment tools can aid the flow and structure and ensure specific information is obtained and or measured. However, it is important to explain if you are going to write notes or complete an assessment tool and to discuss the issue of confidentiality relating to information being shared.[5]

Assessment tools can be disadvantageous, creating a barrier between the patient and professional, taking the focus away from the patient's identified needs or concerns. However, if they are completed with sensitivity, maintaining eye contact, this should not be intrusive to effective communication.

Primary factors of assessment

Assessment is:

- continuous
- ongoing
- detailed.

Eight primary factors can aid focus on points of assessment. By taking these points a picture of the person's story develops that aids further intervention and assessment.

1 Ensure the setting is right:
    - *initial contact* – building trust and a therapeutic relationship
    - *introduction* – friendly, warm, social, negotiation.

2 Person's story – *listen*:
  - *understanding* – the person's perspective
  - *appreciation* – of the person's emotional journey
  - *judgement* – requires good clinical judgement; the person may be poorly, tired and vulnerable
  - *powerful and important* – what the person has to say is integral to them and their illness.
3 What are the primary concerns?
  - *explore* – physical, psychological, spiritual, emotional, economical and social aspects
  - *importance* – what is important to the person?
  - *symptoms* – what is the most troublesome symptom?
  - *directness* – be direct when exploring symptoms.
4 What is the person's understanding of their:
  - *illness/disease* – what does this *mean* for the person?
  - *hopes*
  - *expectations*
  - *ideas*
  - *belief systems*
  - *support*
  - *worries*.
5 Who is important to the person?
  - *support from* – who supports the patient?
  - *support to* – is this person a carer?
6 Exploration of feelings:
  - *illness* – ask 'How does your illness make you feel?'
  - *coping* – ask 'What helps you to cope?'
7 Listen:
  - *attentive* – listen to what is said and what is not said
  - *silence* – do not be afraid to use silence
  - *touch* – use appropriate touch to comfort and reassure
  - *clarify* – feedback and check to clarify and demonstrate your understanding and comprehension
  - *summarise* – bring together and clarify the problems
  - *explain* – offer careful explanation of key points; explain in simple terms, e.g.:
    - what is happening
    - what will happen next
    - medication
    - what are the options.
8 Sexuality:
  - *underacknowledged* – often by the professional
  - *expectation* – patients expect professionals to approach topics of sexuality
  - *sensitivity*:
    - *aim* – not to be intrusive
    - *approach* – use a gentle sensitive approach
    - *demonstrate an openness to discuss* – the person can choose whether or not to respond.

Skills used in assessment

There is a diversity of skills used during assessment. Each patient is unique regardless of lifestyle, religious belief or ethnic group. It is important to believe in the person as an equal human being.[6] The professional should be aware of his or her own values to ensure a non-judgemental approach towards patient and family. The way the assessment is conducted, and information collected, influences the rapport between professional, patient and family. This in turn affects the process of any treatment and interventions that follow.

Non-verbal communications

Use of non-verbal communications assists in demonstrating your interest and attention to the person. During a typical interaction between two people 33% of what is exchanged is verbal and 66% non-verbal. Therefore, it is imperative to:

- maintain a relaxed body posture
- maintain appropriate eye contact
- maintain physical 'openness' – sitting directly facing the patient with your face and body
- lean forward slightly – without invading their personal space
- use appropriate relaxed facial expressions, and occasional smiles
- nod head in encouragement.

Active listening

Listening involves:

- receiving sounds
- accurately understanding their meaning.

To be listened to is therapeutic, without necessarily involving other interactions.[7]

- Be sensitive to vocal cues.
- Listening:
  - assists in creating a relationship – the patient feels heard and understood
  - enables the patient to begin to share his or her *world* with you
  - allows the patient sufficient time to talk and complete statements before asking further questions or making comments.

Silences

Silences may feel uncomfortable. The natural tendency is to break silences by speaking. However, it is important to consider the value of silence for both the patient and professional. Advantages of silence include the following.

- Silence may allow time to collect their – and your – thoughts before continuing.
- The patient may be struggling with strong feelings and the ability to verbalise these.
- Some patients will inevitably be less communicative and require more encouragement to talk.

Encouragement

It is important to encourage communication; this might include:

- using *open* questions – 'How do you feel today?'
- offering verbal encouragement – 'Tell me more about that'
- keeping the focus on their situation
- using your tone of voice to indicate interest.

Clarification of communication

Checking and feeding back your understanding of what has been said demonstrates interest and clarifies meaning and intent:

- use of questions that confirm the patient's meaning is understood – 'What do you mean by that?'
- facilitates the gathering and assimilation of detailed information.

Empathy

To be alongside and demonstrate an understanding of the person's situation and experience is pivotal.

- Use statements to demonstrate understanding from the patient's perspective, assisting the patient to go into more depth.
- Try to be relaxed with natural and spontaneous responses.
- Be sensitive to the person's feelings with the awareness that we are unable to fully understand or appreciate another person's situation. We cannot *fix it*; we can only help the patient to explore it.
- The art of assessment is in the *listening*.

Issues to consider

Case scenario 1.1 highlights some of the issues to be considered in assessment.

Case scenario 1.1

Sid (66) has been feeling unwell for several months with increased shortness of breath and reduced energy levels. After encouragement from his wife he visited his general practitioner (GP). He was referred to a thoracic physician who arranged further investigations. These confirmed a non-small cell cancer of the right lung. Although the cancer was inoperable Sid received a single dose of external palliative radiotherapy to the lung field.

Sid was shocked and expressed anger about the diagnosis, finding it very difficult to come to terms with the poor prognosis and increased limitations on his lifestyle.

Sid and his wife Anne live in a large three-storey house, where he is having difficulties managing the stairs due to increasing shortness of breath and pain which radiates through the chest wall. Sid has been very reluctant to have his bed moved downstairs although has moved into the spare bedroom as he feels he disturbs Anne at night. Sid is reluctant to have an increase of the analgesia, as he feels he will 'lose control' if taking stronger analgesia.

Anne is keen to care for Sid at home although she tells you he tends to vent his feelings of anger and frustration on her verbally, which she finds distressing and difficult to deal with at times. Anne tends to put on a *brave face* when family and professionals visit. Admitting to problems would be 'unfair to Sid'. They have close family relationships with four grown-up children and numerous grandchildren. All live in the local area, visiting frequently to offer their parents both practical and emotional support. Their eldest daughter Jane has been expressing concerns about her father's attitude towards Anne and feels they may not continue to manage at home unless they accept more assistance.

Self-assessment exercise 1.1
Time: 20 minutes

Make a list of problems you've identified.
How could you help?

Assessment of the physical and psychological state for both patient and carers is essential to ensure that appropriate levels of support and treatment interventions can be offered.[8] The information received at referral may be restricted to clinical findings, giving limited or no indication of the patient's main concerns.[9]

Observations

Self-assessment exercise 1.2
Time: 15 minutes

What observations could you make while completing the assessment?

Observations are valuable. By taking into account the patient's general appearance, possible weight loss, skin colour and clear symptoms – e.g. shortness of breath, pain on movement – the professional can gain important supportive insight into the patient's problem. With experience these observations are almost intuitive.

Key tip 1.1

Do not dismiss your intuitive feelings:

- they are there for a reason
- they are telling you something.

Enquire about your observations. Ask further questions regarding physical symptoms, e.g. pain, nausea, bowel habits, sleep pattern, appetite. Establish specific details of symptoms and the medication being taken on a regular basis and the effects of medications. Ask about any mobility limitations. The patient may not think this important or accidentally omit to tell you. Professionals require a knowledge base of symptom management and awareness to be able to interpret this information.[10]

Checking

Check if symptoms are restricting daily living activities, e.g. work, social and leisure time. Experience will assist in alerting the professionals to cues given by the patient, e.g. *'I am not sleeping well.'* This needs to be clarified and the problems established.

Clarify and enable patient's and family understanding

Try to clarify the patient's and family understanding of the expected prognosis. Enable the patient and family to talk about fears and feelings about this with open questions. The feelings may be expressed by anger about the situation, or open emotions with tears and obvious distress. However, do not assume you know what the anger is about. *Ask!* For some it will be a relief to be able to talk openly to someone outside of their family, as they are reluctant to distress them further. Anxiety may also be conveyed by:

- body language
- facial expressions
- fidgeting with their hands
- generalised restlessness.

The family will have their own concerns and fears. It is important to enable the opportunity for them to be expressed too, away from the patient if appropriate. Explore the usual family structure, their relationship with the patient and other family members. *Ask* about the support available, or conflicts there may be between family members. Be mindful that this type of information may not come to light until subsequent visits. Remember that *assessment is a continuous, ongoing process*.

Assessment – an ongoing process

The time taken to complete the assessment is determined by the responsiveness of the patient and the complexity of the situation. It is important that the assessment remain focused. However, time should be allowed for the individual to talk through their issues without feeling hurried.

Seek questions and contributions

Before concluding the assessment it is important to check if the patient or family have any further questions or concerns. At the end of each meeting with patient and family:

- review the main problems as determined by the patient
- set priority for these

- discuss an action plan
- discuss options and interventions
- encourage questions and clarification
- discuss with the patient and family the nature and frequency of further contacts
- ensure the patient and family know how to contact you
- plan for regular reviews
- reinforce any information given
- evaluate changes in the interventions
- liaise with other members of the interdisciplinary team.

Remember some patients will have problems that are long standing; you will be unable to change these, other than offer emotional support and be there when needed. Inevitably there will be the distress of the illness for the patient, family and all their friends.

Assessment and cultural considerations[11]

Any individual – regardless of race, culture, colour, creed, social and/or economic status – has the right to expect and receive appropriate treatment and interventions. For some, the lack of adequate cultural knowledge will prevent proper interactions taking place in any meaningful way. The issue of transcultural health and social care is broad. In this section, we look at some of the problems and difficulties encountered by the patient and family when seeking treatment and intervention.

As well as attending to the patient and family history, the professional needs to assess the issues related to migration and culture. If ignored, the individual's racial and cultural identity is rebuffed. It is a mistake to assume that, by treating an individual from an ethnic minority as one would any other patient, adequate treatment and intervention will be provided. Moreover, the professional may deal with the patient and family as a *cultural stereotype*. Such an approach ignores the social and interpersonal factors that are relevant in assessment. This often results from the professional being overwhelmed by unfamiliar racial and cultural characteristics.

Another difficult area relates to differences in the presentation of physical, emotional, spiritual, social and psychological problems. Where there are language difficulties, an interpreter should be used. The interpreter, however, must be carefully selected. If s/he is not from any of the caring professions, there may be difficulty explaining information or asking questions in a meaningful way. Equally, if the interpreter is a member of the patient's family, this can lead to embarrassment.

Some examples follow of how references and beliefs can be misinterpreted through a lack of knowledge on cultural issues.

- When a Pakistani refers to himself as being 'Royal', s/he is not necessarily deluded; it means simply that s/he comes from a wealthy family. This is not a grandiose delusion in cultural terms.
- *'The good lord is talking to me'* is an expression often used by Afro-Caribbean people of religious background. This can mistakenly be perceived as the client experiencing auditory hallucinations.

Building a rapport requires time, patience, tolerance and perseverance. The patient and/or family may be reluctant to allow a cultural outsider to get too close. The style of questioning adopted by Western society often does not fit the conceptual models used in other cultures. The professional who insists on using this style of questioning may lose credibility in that s/he may be perceived as ignorant. This makes it difficult to facilitate participation and involvement in treatment and intervention planning. On the other hand, members of other cultures often expect the professional to have all the answers.

Interventions and treatment should be as free from trauma as possible. Patients and family from a minority culture are often at a disadvantage in a system designed for white Europeans. To conclude this section there follows a list of *dos and do nots* (Box 1.1), that applies to all cultures. The list is not exhaustive; it is anticipated that it will be used as a reference when involved in the treatment and interventions with the individual from all cultures.

Box 1.1   Cultural considerations – dos and do-nots[11]

Name

- *Do not:*
  - use Western titles, e.g. Mr, Miss, Ms, Mrs
  - ask non-Christians for a Christian name.
- *Do:*
  - ask for family name or first name
  - avoid repetition in clinical notes; find out the correct family name first rather than misuse several differing names.

Language

- *Do not:*
  - assume that all ethnic groups speak English
  - assume that all minority ethnic groups do not speak English
  - use the family to interpret intimate questions
  - use the family to break bad news; s/he may avoid the issue if it is believed to be too stressful for the patient.
- *Do:*
  - avoid making assumptions by using accurate assessment procedures
  - use an interpreter who understands medical terminology; this will avoid stress for the interpreter, patient and family and avoid misinterpretation
  - be aware that women may only ask intimate questions of women in some cultures; this avoids wrong information being passed, and embarrassment.

Religion

- *Do not:*
  - generalise about the patient and family religion
  - mistake religious objects or symbols for jewellery.
- *Do:*
  - remember that for Buddhists, Christians, Jews, Sikhs, Hindus and Muslims, religion may be an integral part of daily life

- avoid incorrect assumptions; find out the different beliefs and approaches
- record clearly and make note of the patient and family wish to see or have present a representative from their religion
- ask the family if the patient is not able to relay this to you
- remember that many Eastern religions fast on certain days; pray at certain times; wear religious object or symbols
- check if treatment or interventions will compromise any religious beliefs
- inform the patient and family of any treatment or interventions, before commencing, to check religious beliefs
- check religious observations with the patient and family
- consult with religious advisors or teachers to gain permission and/or to obtain exemption, to allow procedures to take place; ensure s/he explains this to the patient and family.

Diet

- *Do not:*
  - give Jews or Muslims pork or pork products.
- *Do:*
  - make sure that other meat offered to Muslims has been religiously slaughtered by the halal method (naturally slaughtered)
  - remember that not all Jewish people eat kosher food (specially prepared to make pure)
  - remember that not all Muslims eat halal meat
  - consult the patient and family about any diet preferences
  - remember that meal times are family occasions in Eastern culture; matters relating to the family are often discussed here
  - remember that being taken out of a close family environment can be frightening and cause loneliness, which may in turn cause loss of appetite
  - invite the family to bring food and join in meal times, if at all possible and practical; if it is not, explain why.

Personal hygiene

- *Do:*
  - remember that to Sikhs, Hindus and Muslims, washing in still water is considered unclean
  - supply the patient with a jug of water and bowl and/or running tap and empty wash-basin to allow hand, face and body washing
  - make exceptions if the patient is dependent
  - remember that Muslims use the *right hand* for eating and food preparation, and the *left hand* for self-cleansing and other procedures; anyone unable to do this because of injury or health reasons will need counselling and discussion relating to ways of surmounting this problem (it may be useful to supply plastic gloves).

Modesty

- *Do not:*
  - compromise the patient's dignity and modesty.

- *Do:*
  - remember that exposure of the female body to a male will cause distress in certain cultures, especially if the patient is in *purdah* (the duration of menstruation)
  - offer separate bays in mixed bedded wards or, if possible, a single room, especially for the patient in *purdah*
  - remember that hospital gowns expose more than they cover, and therefore are often unacceptable
  - avoid exposure of arms or legs; add additional covering to protect modesty.

Skin and hair

- *Do:*
  - remember that Afro hair may be brittle or dry; add moisturiser or oil to the scalp and comb regularly
  - remember to ask the patient what s/he uses for skin moisturiser
  - remember that dark-skinned people are prone to keloid scarring (hyper-keratinisation); invasive treatment will cause excessive pigmented scarring
  - remember to inject or undertake invasive procedures in a site that will avoid disfigurement if possible.

Hospital procedures

- *Do not:*
  - give Jehovah's Witnesses blood transfusions
  - give Muslims, Jews and vegetarians iron injections derived from pigs
  - give insulin of bovine origin to Hindus or Sikhs
  - give insulin of porcine origin to Jews or Muslims.
- *Do:*
  - give careful thought to procedures and routines before commencing them
  - remember that discussion of elimination or other intimate issues may be culturally offensive
  - approach all patients sensitively, ensure privacy, and maintain the individual's right to self-respect
  - remember that some medications, interventions and treatments may be taboo for some religious groups
  - remember that some medications have an alcohol base which may be forbidden in some cultural groups
  - remember that the patient with an alcohol problem may wish to avoid alcohol-based preparations
  - be aware of all preparations likely to contain potentially taboo or offensive ingredients.

Visiting

- *Do:*
  - remember that limiting visiting to two people may cause distress in extended family cultures
  - remember West Indian, Asian and Middle Eastern families like to visit as a family

- remember that the *family* may include children, uncles, aunts, grand-children, parents and grandparents
- compromise over visiting, and numbers visiting per bed, if possible
- remember that open visiting can be more accommodating
- allow the family to participate in the patient's care.

Myths

- *Do not:*
  - believe that people from different races have a low pain threshold; this is incorrect, e.g.
    - Japanese people may smile or laugh when in pain, thus avoiding loss of face
    - Anglo-Saxons may be sullen and withdrawn, portraying the stiff-upper-lip image
    - Eastern Europeans, Greeks, and Italians express pain vocally and freely.
- *Do:*
  - remember that every individual has a different level of pain tolerance, regardless of race, culture of origin or creed.

Death and bereavement

- *Do not:*
  - deny the family the right to participate in last offices as this will increase the pain already being experienced and may slow down the grieving process.
- *Do:*
  - involve the patient and family in the care
  - remember that Eastern cultures like to take an active part in the care of the dying relative, especially last offices
  - remember that in certain cultures, custom and practice will need to be followed if the patient is to proceed along the continuum of life following his or her earthly death
  - ensure that you are fully conversant with specific cultural require-ments for death, bereavement and last offices
  - negotiate to minimise anxiety and allow some participation, when the family's wishes come into conflict with hospital policies and pro-cedures; this will assist the grieving process
  - compromise; the patient and family have only one chance to say their goodbyes.

Conclusion

The nature of assessment must vary to suit the circumstances. The prime focus will be the illness, although this needs to be understood in context with the patient's life, beliefs and values. Rather than seeing assessment as the professional collecting information and forming clinical judgements, it is accurate to think of the patient, family and professional jointly assessing the problems and considering possible solutions.

As professionals working in palliative care, we are privileged to encounter people at a distressful time in their lives. This requires an individual approach, using sensitivity and skills to complete an assessment before being able to initiate an action plan and appropriate interventions.

References

1   Mason P. Essentials of assessment. In: Cooper DB, editor. *Alcohol Use*. Oxford: Radcliffe Medical Press; 2000, Chapter 14, pp. 162–163.
2   Lugton J. *Communicating with Dying People and Their Relatives*. Oxford: Radcliffe Medical Press; 2002.
3   Montgomery Dossey B. *Holistic Nursing: a hand book for practice*. New York: Aspen Publishing Inc; 1995.
4   Department of Health. *The Expert Patient: a new approach to chronic disease management in the 21st century*. London: Stationery Office; 2001.
5   Faulkner A, Maguire P. *Talking to Cancer Patients and Their Relatives*. Oxford: Oxford University Press; 1994.
6   Davies B, Oberle K. Dimensions of the supportive role of the nurse in palliative care. *Oncology Nursing Forum*. 1990; **17**(1): 87–94.
7   Nelson-Jones R. *Practical Counselling and Helping Skills*, 2nd edition. London: Cassell; 1990.
8   Mirando S. Palliative care needs assessment. *International Journal of Palliative Nursing*. 2004; **10**(12): 602–604.
9   Luker K, Austen L, Caress A *et al*. The importance of 'knowing the patient': community nurses' constructions of quality in proving palliative care. *Journal of Advanced Nursing*. 2000; **31**(4): 755–782.
10 Davies J, McVicar A. Issues in effective pain control from assessment to management. *International Journal of Palliative Nursing*. 2000; **6**(4): 162–169.
11 Cooper DB. Transcultural issues and approaches. In: Wright H, Giddey M, editors. *Mental Health Nursing: from first principle to professional practice*. London: Chapman and Hall; 1993, pp. 191–201.

To learn more

• Baille L. Empathy in the nurse patient relationship. *Nursing Times*. 1995; **9**(20): 29–32.
• Lugton J. *Communicating with Dying People and Their Relatives*. Oxford: Radcliffe Medical Press; 2002.
• Maguire P, Pitceathly C. Key communication skills and how to acquire them. *British Medical Journal*. 2002; **325**: 697–700.
• Nelson- Jones R. *Practical Counselling and Helping Skills*, 2nd edition. London: Cassell; 1990.
• Oliviere D, Hargreaves R, Monroe B. *Good Practice in Palliative Care*. Aldershot: Ashgate; 1998.
• Purnell LD, Paulanka BJ. *Transcultural Health Care: a culturally competent approach*, 2nd edition. Philadelphia: FA Davis Company; 2003.

Complementary chapters

See also Stepping into Palliative Care 1: relationships and responses

- Chapter 2: What is palliative care?
- Chapter 3: The cancer journey
- Chapter 4: The experience of illness
- Chapter 5: The psychological impact of serious illness
- Chapter 6: Hope and coping strategies
- Chapter 7: The therapeutic relationship
- Chapter 8: Gold Standards Framework: a programme for community palliative care
- Chapter 9: Integrated care pathways
- Chapter 11: The value of teamwork
- Chapter 13: Communication: the essence of good practice, management and leadership
- Chapter 15: Transcultural and ethnic issues at the end of life
- Chapter 16: Sexuality and palliative care

Chapter 2

Introduction to pain management

Trevor Mitten

Pre-reading exercise 2.1
Time: 25 minutes

- What questions could you ask the patient about his or her pain?
- Have you used a pain assessment scale to assess pain in patients?
  - Which one did you use?
  - Why?
  - Is there a better one available for your patient group?
- Think of a time you, or someone close to you, were experiencing pain.
  - What steps did you take to identify the cause of the pain and to manage it?

Review your answers at the end of this chapter to see if you explored all approaches, or if you could have achieved more effective pain management.

Primary aims of pain management

- A good night's sleep.
- Relief at rest.
- Relief on movement – although this may be more difficult to achieve.

Assessing pain

In pain management, the single most important factors are:

- ask the *right* questions
- *listen* to the answers.

The primary function of pain assessment is to ensure that the patient, family and professional understands:

- what is said
- what is not said.

Therefore, the prerequisite for good pain management is a full and comprehensive assessment and history.

One sentence can make a clear connection between:

- what the patient is feeling
- the type of pain experienced.

To do this we must *really listen* to what is being said and *observe* body language, which is an important indicator when assessing pain.

Close observation of body language, and expressions relating to disruption of the patient's normal activity, reveal as much about the presence and nature of pain as the description of the pain itself. This may include:

- complaints of waking at night with discomfort
- sitting in a 'special chair' – it is common for people in pain to seek a chair that is perceived to reduce pain levels
- propping with cushions
- leaning into the pain
- use of the hand or other object(s) to apply pressure at the pain site
- constant rubbing of pain site.

An essential aid to pain assessment is the family. It is imperative that family views are sought and taken into account. The patient may not wish to be seen as complaining or weak; therefore, pain may be under-reported. Moreover, it is not uncommon for pain to be 'eased' or to disappear altogether during conversation with the professional.

The individual may experience *referred* pain in one area that originates from elsewhere. It is estimated that up to 25% of cancer sufferers have four or more pains.[1] Therefore, it is important to ask if the individual is experiencing different types of pain, as they may well have more than one. Equally, the pain experienced might not be directly related to the cancer, although it is important to address all pain.

Ongoing assessment and evaluation of pain is pivotal: a continuum, not a one-off exercise. It may be that as one pain is managed the individual becomes aware of another. Pain may also reappear later and/or become transformed into a different type of pain.

Assessment tools

The use of pain diaries or pain assessment tools is an important part of assessment, and gives the patient a sense of control. Rating mechanisms include:

- visual analogue scale
- numerical rating scale
- The London Hospital pain observation chart[2] – the individual draws the pain site on a body outline.

Pain assessment in groups such as cognitively impaired older adults can be difficult to assess and this can result in poor management and outcomes.[3] Examples of assessment in this group include:

- Abbey pain scale – a structured pain-assessment scale in end-stage dementia.[3]
- Doloplus 2 – a scale for elderly patients with verbal communication disorder.[4]

However, while assessment tools have a valuable role, they are not effective in isolation and should form part of a full oral and visual assessment.

Assessing the unconscious patient

Relatives often ask how we can tell if someone unconscious is in pain. The signs can include:

- restlessness
- frowning
- tachycardia.

This can be contrasted with the 'groaning' breathing sometimes evident in the last few hours, where the individual is not in pain, but has noisy respiration.

Pain awareness

Terminology is important. A patient may deny pain. This may be because of adaptation to chronic pain: the individual is unable to acknowledge or verbalise its presence. It is common for patients to describe pain in terms of *discomfort* rather than directly to describe it as pain. By asking the patient if s/he has discomfort or an ache, pain may be acknowledged. Therefore, this should not be ignored but explored carefully with the patient and family.

Even though individuals' reports of pain are accepted as the most reliable indicator of how much pain is experienced, nurses tend not to rely on self-reporting.[5] If effective intervention in pain management is to be achieved we must acknowledge that the patient knows his or her own body more than anyone else, and accept that s/he holds the key to the problem of pain.

Breakthrough pain

Breakthrough pain is an increase of pain which *spikes* above a baseline of controlled pain, where pain can increase markedly and needs immediate quick-acting analgesia – sometimes referred to as a *rescue dose* – to reduce the pain (*see* Figure 2.1).

Rapidly increasing pain

Rapid increase in pain levels may be experienced. This often occurs during the final stages of life, and is frightening for the patient and family, often causing feelings of anxiety and panic. Prompt review, a calm manner and appropriate intervention may help to allay fears and concerns. The importance of awareness that such situations can arise, and that they require prompt, effective management, cannot be overemphasised.

Analgesia may need to be increased rapidly, especially as the situation can change within the hour. Some professionals express concern at how quickly the need for pain relief increases. This can be a source of anxiety for the professional. The need for analgesia during terminal illness is often considerably greater than the level of

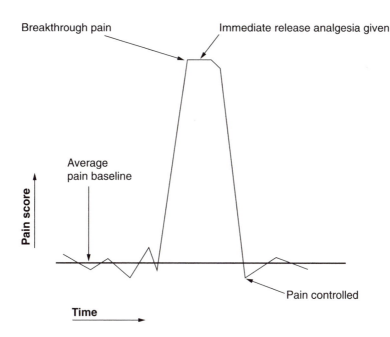

Figure 2.1   Breakthrough pain.

analgesia recommended by the professional on a routine basis. There is no good reason for withholding adequate analgesia. Discussion within the interdisciplinary team will help to support the professional.

Simple measures

Often the professional finds that the focus is on medication, which is perceived as a panacea for the relief of pain. Nevertheless, simple measures can often be effective in pain control. Simple measures are non-invasive, readily available and most importantly empower the individual or carer to feel they can do something to lessen suffering themselves. Simple measure include:

- careful positioning and judicious use of pillows
- heat therapy:
  - hot bath
  - wheat bag – check for allergies first as some people may develop an allergic reaction to the wheat or the bags may be impregnated with aromatherapy oils[6]
- massage
- movement – changing position of simple movements can help to reduce positional pain.

Key tip 2.1

- Not all pain can be completely relieved.
- It is important that we are able to support people through their pain.

Compliance with treatment

For pain relief to be effective, it is essential to adequately explain the need for analgesia. Allowing time for discussion is essential in order to allay fears and maximise compliance with medication.

Some individuals fear morphine dependency. In many cases, the patient who is receiving high-dose opioids can effectively reduce medication following treatment, e.g. radiotherapy or nerve blocks, with little or no effect.[7] One reason for deferred prescribing of morphine is the concern that *tolerance* may develop. However, the need for an increased dosage of opioids is associated with disease progression rather than pharmacological tolerance.[7,8] This should be fully explained to the patient and family.

Analgesic ladder

The World Health Organization (WHO) analgesic ladder[9] is a useful guide to prescription of the appropriate level of analgesia (*see* Figure 2.2). This progresses from Step 1, when the use of non-opioids, e.g. paracetamol and non-steroidal anti-inflammatory drugs (NSAIDs – e.g. ibuprofen) may be appropriate. If the pain remains uncontrolled, although the maximum dose has been achieved, then progression to Step 2 follows. A weak opioid, e.g. co-codamol or dihydrocodeine, with NSAIDs and other adjuvants, as appropriate, may be effective. After the maximum dose of Step 2 drugs has been reached, then progression to Step 3 is recommended. Step 3 drugs include the strong opioids, e.g. morphine, prescribed with or without adjuvant drugs.

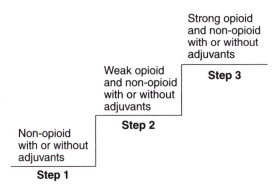

Figure 2.2   WHO three-step ladder.

Key tip 2.2

- Adjuvant drugs are used to complement other drugs and to maximise pain relief.
- They can be used at any step of the analgesic ladder.

A stumbling block

The main problem with prescribing analgesics is a reluctance in moving from level-2 to level-3 drugs. Professionals, patient and family appear concerned about morphine and describe the pain as *'not that bad yet'*, when faced with a choice of progression to such drugs. However, if the maximum dose of a level-2 drug is achieved without effect, there is little evidence to suggest replacing this with another level-2 drug. Level 3 is the logical progression if pain management is to be effective.

Key tip 2.3

- The WHO analgesic ladder is merely a guide to pain management. It is neither essential, nor necessary, to follow the ladder in all cases.
- For some patients it may be more appropriate to prescribe Step-3 drugs immediately – hence the need for a thorough assessment of pain.

Opioids in pain management

There are multiple liquid morphines. The most common of these is Oramorph solution. This is absorbed quickly (*peak plasma concentration is 30 mins*),[10] and is useful for breakthrough pain, or to assess opioid need *prior* to switching to a long-acting formulation.

Oral morphine

- Strong opioid of choice for cancer.
- Regular laxative should be prescribed whenever morphine is used; constipation almost inevitably occurs.
- Initially an anti-emetic may be needed if nausea or vomiting is a problem.
- Sedation can be a problem with large doses, though the individual does adapt to the increased dose and becomes less sedated after 3–4 days. This can recur with each dose increase.
- Regular use of morphine is much more effective than *as required* doses.[11]
- Standard strengths are:
  - 10 mg/5 ml
  - 100 mg/5 ml (dyed pink).
- Tastes sharp but can be sweetened with a little neat blackcurrant cordial.

Key tip 2.4

Oral morphine – use of quick-acting preparations

- Commence morphine using a quick-acting liquid or tablet before switching to sustained-release morphine.
- Enables rapid titration to the therapeutic level.
- Oral rescue doses of liquid morphine can be offered every 30 minutes in extreme cases.[12]

Sublingual

The administration of sublingual Oramorph can be used in terminal stages. It may be considered where remote location or lack of other medications precludes other alternatives. There are also single dose, twist-top, plastic vial preparations of Oramorph (unit dose vials) available in strengths:

- 10 mg/5 ml
- 30 mg/5 ml
- 100 mg/5 ml.

The single dose twist is effective where a person lacks the manual dexterity to measure using a spoon or syringe. In addition, they are useful when travelling, and can be squirted straight in the mouth. There is also a tablet form of quick-release morphine called Sevredol, available as 10 mg, 20 mg and 50 mg.

Breakthrough pain

Oral doses for breakthrough pain can be offered every 60–90 minutes as appropriate.[13] The rescue dose for breakthrough pain is one-third of the 12-hourly dose of sustained-release morphine. It is important to review the effect of the morphine and the pain regularly. The dose should be increased as appropriate, taking into account all of the rescue doses taken within a 24-hour period. If additional doses are required several times during the day, this suggests that the regular dose needs to be increased.[1]

Key tip 2.5

When pain is problematic at night, waking the patient, increase the dose of Oramorph at bedtime.

Morphine sulphate tablets (MST) in a sustained-release formulation are available in 5 mg, 10 mg, 15 mg, 30 mg, 60 mg, 100 mg and 200 mg, and are suitable for twice-daily administration. If pain is not relieved by 90% after 24 hours, increase the dose[1] e.g. from:

- 5 to 10 mg
- 10 to 15 mg
- 20 to 30 mg.

In addition, consider adjuvant drugs when administering strong opioids.

Key tip 2.6

Different types of pain, e.g. bone or nerve pain, respond to different types of medication.

Opioid preparations

There are several long- and short-acting opioid preparations, summarised in Table 2.1.

Prescribing consideration

Consideration must be given to possible side effects related to opioid use (*see* Table 2.2). These may include:

- *possible toxic effects*
- *intolerable side effects* – constipation, nausea, vomiting, sedation – which may outweigh the benefits
- *renal failure* – accumulation of morphine metabolites decreasing effectiveness of a strong opioid; switching to an alternative strong opioid may reduce this effect – this is referred to as *rotation of opioids*[14]
- *compliance* – fear of the drug and an unwillingness to take morphine. Alternative opioids may elicit compliance.

Diamorphine profile

- Chemically, diamorphine consists of two morphine molecules locked together.
- It is the preferred drug of choice for use in a syringe driver for subcutaneous infusion.
- It has a much higher solubility in solutions.
- It is twice as potent as morphine when administered by injection.[15]

Converting from morphine to diamorphine

When converting from *morphine* to *diamorphine*, the following factors will need to be considered.[1]

- When converting from *oral morphine* to *subcutaneous diamorphine*, divide the 24-hour *oral morphine* dose by three.
- Increments in dose should be in the range 25–50%.
- Additional subcutaneous doses for breakthrough pain are calculated as *one-sixth* of the 24-hour dose.[15]

Table 2.1 Opioid preparations

Drug	Starting dose	Indications for use
Fentanyl transmucosal lozenge on a stick (Actiq)	200 micrograms repeated after 15 minutes if pain unrelieved	For rapid relief of incident or breakthrough pain. Good for those unable to take oral medication
Fentanyl TTS, transdermal patch (fentanyl patch)	12–25 micrograms every 72 hours	Stable severe pain
Hydromorphone	4 mg 12-hourly	Can be opened and sprinkled on to soft, cold food
Methadone	Specialist advice is needed pre-prescription	Used for severe pain, intractable cough, and opioid rotation. It has a long half-life in the body (i.e. it takes a long time to be broken down), and can accumulate to toxic levels (*seek specialist advice*). May be beneficial for neuropathic pain. As an opioid rotation agent it has a higher delta-receptor effect than morphine, and a wide spectrum of activity. For cough a dose of 2–4 mg at night or twice daily may help
Morcap	20 mg once a day (licensed for 12-hourly administration)	This is a capsule form of morphine that can be opened and sprinkled onto food
MST suspension	10–30 mg twice a day for opioid-naive patients or those previously on weak opioids	MST suspension is a sachet of powder which, when mixed with water, forms a suspension that the patient drinks. This is useful if swallowing tablets is a problem. It can also be syringed down a gastrostomy tube. It is available in a variety of doses up to 200 mg sachet but is difficult to mix without forming lumps. To ensure even distribution of the mix use 10–20 ml of very hot water as the base, and sprinkle the powder on slowly while stirring gently. Ensure the mix is cool before administration
MXL	30 mg once a day	This is a once-daily capsule preparation of sustained-release morphine
Oramorph	10–30 mg 4-hourly as needed	Useful for breakthrough pain. Absorbed quickly
Oxycodone	30 mg suppository 8-hourly	Useful for patients who are unable to tolerate oral medication. This is given as a suppository, providing 6–8 hours of relief. Useful if unable to take orally and a syringe driver is inappropriate
Oxycodone	10 mg twice daily	Lasts 12 hours
Oxynorm	Capsules 5 mg Liquid 5 mg/5 ml	Both immediate release last 4–6 hours
Sevredol	10–30 mg 4-hourly	Used for breakthrough pain. Immediate release morphine in tablet form

Table 2.2 Morphine side effects

Side effect	Treatment
Constipation	Laxatives, e.g. • co-danthramer • senna • docusate.
Nausea/vomiting	Anti-emetics: • haloperidol • metoclopramide. *Often passes off after a few days so need to review.*
Drowsiness	Wears off after a few days but may recur temporarily after dose increase.
Bad dreams/hallucinations	• Not that common, assessment of opioid toxicity. • Reduce dose. • Add antipsychotic, e.g. haloperidol 1.5 mg tds. • Switch to different strong opioid.

OxyContin – prolonged release oxycodone hydrochloride

A long-acting 12-hourly oxycodone tablet (*OxyContin*) is twice as potent as morphine. 10 mg oral *OxyContin* is approximately equivalent to 20 mg oral morphine. There are a wide range of 12-hourly strengths. The usual starting dose is:

- 10 mg 12-hourly – dependent on pain severity and previous history of analgesic requirements
- 5 mg 12-hourly – titration or those patients who might be susceptible to opioid-related side effect. Titration is in increments of 25–50% until pain relief is achieved.

Other 12-hourly strengths include:

- 20 mg
- 40 mg
- 80 mg.

An immediate relief quick-acting liquid or tablet form (*oxynorm*) is available.[16] There is also a rectal preparation – *oxycodone suppositories*.

Fentanyl

The transdermal patch *(Durogesic D-Trans, fentanyl)* is a clear sticky patch, applied to the skin, that normally lasts 3 days. Durogesic D-Trans is smaller and adheres better than previous patches. Fentanyl patches may cause less constipation and the daytime somnolence caused by morphine.[17] Transdermal patches are in five strengths:

- 12 microgram
- 25 microgram

- 50 microgram
- 75 microgram
- 100 microgram.

A patch will provide good pain relief, and seem less *medical* and intrusive than the subcutaneous route. If a patch is already in place it is unwise to switch to another strong opioid at the end of life[18] unless pain is increasing, as the crossover period may lead to pain breakthrough.

Essential knowledge for fentanyl patch preparation

- Fentanyl can take from 12 to 24 hours to achieve maximum blood concentration.[11]
- If the patient is currently receiving morphine sulphate tablets (MST), the fentanyl patch is applied with the last oral dose of MST.[19]
- Fentanyl patches are not suitable if pain is escalating rapidly due to slow absorption rate.
- It is essential that patients with fentanyl patches are prescribed quick-release opioids for breakthrough pain:
  – this must be given in the correct dose for the patch size
  – the dose should be increased whenever the patch size is increased.
- Some reports have indicated that the fentanyl patch only lasts for 2 days[20] – *the normal application period is 3 days*. If pain control is maximised at 2 days but decreases on day 3, consider increase in patch strength.
- Continual review of pain is pivotal.
- Counselling is essential for the patient and family throughout.
- Verbal and written guidance about the application of the patch is essential.
- Careful explanation of the potential side effects will ease anxiety and aid compliance.
- Patients *do* find the patches advantageous as the:
  – need for oral medication is reduced
  – comfort is increased
  – daily reminder relating to health may be decreased.
- The normal starting dose is 12 microgram to 25 microgram patch. If the patient is converting from 4-hourly *oral morphine* to *fentanyl*, the *morphine* should be *continued for 12 hours* while the blood concentration achieves maximum saturation.
- For breakthrough pain, *divide the fentanyl patch by 5* (patch/5) to give the *dose in milligrams of diamorphine administered subcutaneously.*[21]

Side effects

A small number of patients experience side effects in the first 24 hours when switching from morphine to fentanyl patches.[19] These can include:

- sweating
- diarrhoea
- bowel cramps
- nausea
- restlessness.

Treatment

One or two doses of oral morphine will give quick release of side effects.

Other fentanyl preparations

- *Transmucosal lozenge on a stick – for rapid reduction of breakthrough pain.* The transmucosal lozenge on a stick (Actiq) is impregnated with a specific strength of fentanyl. This is rolled around the oral mucosa (use artificial saliva spray for a dry mouth). The drug is absorbed across the oral mucosa and is effective after 5 minutes, and for up to 2 hours.[19] The starting dose is always 200 micrograms regardless of the size of the fentanyl patch. Doses are titrated up as necessary. *Continued review is paramount. S*afe and effective, the transmucosal lozenge has advantages over other opioids due to its rapid onset and short duration of action.[19,22]
- *Intravenous injection (alfentanyl)* – good in renal failure.
- *Subcutaneously via syringe driver (alfentanyl)* – for morphine intolerance.

Topical opioids

Topical opioids in a carrier gel (intrasite or metronidazole) for wound pain can be beneficial.[23–25] Topical opioids:

- can be helpful for a wound, e.g. pressure ulcer
- co-jointly with systemic opioids.[26]

One regimen is *1 mg of diamorphine to 1 mg of intrasite gel* applied once daily.[27] Another is in the use of *diamorphine and Instillagel local anaesthetic gel*, or with KY Jelly.[28]

Key tip 2.7

- Fear of seeing the wound may heighten perceived pain.[25]
- Minimise the patient's exposure to seeing the wound during dressing changes – unless otherwise requested by the patient.

Does adding a second opioid improve pain relief?

Inadequate pain management, with escalating opioid doses, in the presence of dose-limiting toxic effects, including

- hallucinations
- confusion
- hyperalgesia
- myoclonus
- sedation
- nausea

may be a problem in some cases. When the patient requires increasing doses of a strong analgesic, benefit may be obtained from using two opioids.[29]

Recent data suggest a possible use of an opioid combination to improve analgesia. A study assessed the effects of adding a second opioid, at low doses, in patients with poor analgesic benefit after dose escalation. A reduction in pain intensity was found by combining two opioids, targeting different sets of *mu* receptors. Observations need to be confirmed in further studies.[29]

Opioid-unresponsive pain

Some pains not fully responsive to opioids include:

1 *Musculoskeletal* – bone pain.
   - Typical description:
     - aching joints – sometimes described as toothache
     - a pressure
     - heaviness in the bone – may be experienced in the back or hip – often worse on movement.
2 *Neurogenic* – nerve pain.
   - Typical description:
     - stabbing
     - shooting
     - burning
     - pins and needles
     - increased sensitivity of skin
     - change in sensation.

Careful and attentive listening to the patient or family's description of the pain provides vital information relating to pain type.

Musculoskeletal – bone pain

Bone pain may arise for a variety of reasons, including:

- osteoarthritis
- pathological fracture
- bone metastases.

Cancers that are likely to cause bone metastases include:

- breast
- prostate
- multiple myeloma
- bronchus
- kidney.

The first-line drugs of choice are non-steroidal anti-inflammatory drugs (NSAIDs). Because of the anti-inflammatory effect, NSAIDs are useful for metastatic bone and soft tissue pains. They can be used with a strong opioid[1] (*see* Table 2.3).

Table 2.3 Anti-inflammatory drugs

Drug	Dose
Aspirin	600 mg four times a day
Ibuprofen	200–600 mg three times a day or brufen retard two tablets daily (800 mg)
Flurbiprofen (Froben)	50–100 mg three times a day – also available as 100 mg suppositories
Diclofenac (Voltarol)	• Oral – 50 mg tds • Oral – 75 mg bd • Suppositories 100 mg
Ketorolac (Toradol)	• Oral – 10 mg tds • Subcutaneous infusion – 60–120 mg over 24 hours
Piroxicam (Feldene)	• Oral – 20 mg od
Feldene melt	• Dissolve on tongue
Diclofenac with misoprostol (arthrotec)	One tablet (50 mg/200 micrograms) tds or one tablet (75 mg/200 micrograms) bd

Essential knowledge for NSAID preparations

- NSAIDs help to control bone pain in 80% of patients.[30]
- It is worth rotating to different non-steroidal drugs if one particular drug does not work.[31]
- Ketorolac is an NSAID which is available in tablet form (10 mg tds–qds)[16] or by intravenous or subcutaneous injection.[32]
  - Administration via a syringe driver is beneficial if other oral NSAIDs have failed.[33] This can be attributed to ketorolac's dual anti-inflammatory and analgesic effect.[34] The improved absorption via the parenteral route also plays a role.
- NSAIDs may cause gastric irritation. A gastroprotective (e.g. omeprazole 20 mg) should be considered.[35]

Bisphosphonates

The use of bisphosphonates in cases of bone pain is encouraging.[36] Even when individuals have a normal calcium level,[37] treatment with a bisphosphonates (e.g. pamidronate 60–90 mg IV every 4–6 weeks) can markedly reduce bone metastases pain. A once-a-day preparation of a bisphosphonate tablet – ibandronate (Bondronat)[38,39] – eliminates the need for hospitalisation for an infusion.

Radiotherapy

- Radiation can reduce pain in 90% of patients with bone pain.[40]
- Radiotherapy can be helpful in reducing pain from bone metastasis.
- A single dose often completes the treatment.

Strontium

- Injections of strontium 89® for the relief of metastatic bone pain is indicated for patients with prostate or breast cancer.[41]
- Strontium follows the pathway of calcium, delivering local radiotherapy to site of bone metastases.

Neurogenic – nerve pain

Nerve pain often follows nerve pathways, e.g. the facial nerve (trigeminal neuralgia) or thoracic nerve (shingles). It is not fully controlled by opioids,[42] but often responds well to antidepressant medication (e.g. *amitriptyline, venlafaxine* – particularly if the sensation is *burning*). Alternatively, anti-epileptic medication – e.g. gabapentin[43] or pregabalin[44] – can be considered (*see* Table 2.4).

Table 2.4 Drug management of neurogenic pain

Drug	Dosage/side effects
Amitriptyline	• 10–75 mg nocte • Can cause dry mouth, blurred vision, sedation
Venlafaxine	• 37.5 mg bd • Increase to 75 mg after 1 week if necessary • Can cause dizziness, dry mouth, insomnia, constipation
Sertraline	• 50–150 mg once daily in the morning • Nausea a problem initially. Also diarrhoea, restlessness, headache
Gabapentin	• 100 mg–600 mg tds – slowly titrated • Can cause dizziness, sedation, nausea, blurred vision
Pregabalin	• 75 mg–300 mg bd • Can cause dizziness, sedation, peripheral oedema

Other treatments for nerve pain

- Epidural/ intrathecal injection.
- Coeliac plexus block.
- Chemical nerve destruction with phenol.
- Surgical nerve destruction (e.g. cordotomy).

The flow chart on opioid-unresponsive pain indicates considerations and actions for addressing these types of pain (*see* Figure 2.3).

Steroids in pain management

The use of steroids in pain management needs to be weighed against the side effects. However, steroids can be effective used appropriately. Steroids are indicated in the following:[19]

- raised intracranial pressure
- spinal cord compression

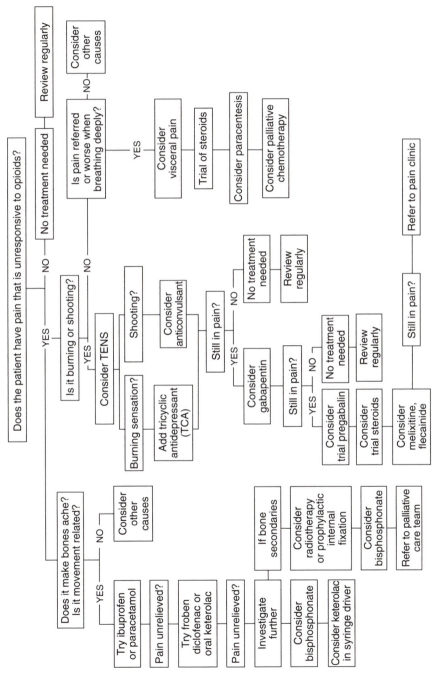

Figure 2.3 Flow chart for opioid-unresponsive pain.

- bone pain
- liver capsule stretch.

Steroid use in symptom palliation

- Reduces cerebral oedema in cerebral tumours/secondaries.
- Lowers raised intracranial pressure.
- Stimulates appetite.
- Provides euphoria and energy for special event, e.g. a wedding.
- Reduces liver capsule pain due to stretching of the viscera.
- Reduces nerve pain by relieving nerve compression or irritation.

Prescribing and administering steroids

Dexamethasone:

- is often the steroid of choice
- is approximately seven times more potent than prednisolone,[19] therefore fewer tablets are needed
- crosses the blood–brain barrier and is useful for patients with cerebral tumours
- tablets can be crushed and made into a suspension with warm water, for ease of swallowing
- is supplied as a sugar-free solution (Dexsol).[45]

To prevent dyspepsia/ulcers a proton pump inhibitor (PPI) or H2 antagonist or misoprostol 200 micrograms helps protect the stomach.

Side effects of steroids

- Gastric irritation or ulceration.
- Water retention.
- Fluid imbalance.
- Immunosuppression.
- Steroid psychosis.
- Oral candidiasis.
- Insomnia.
- Thinning of the skin.
- Hypertension.
- Steroid-induced diabetes.
- Osteoporosis.
- Myopathy.

Key tip 2.8

- Steroids given four times a day can cause nocturnal insomnia.
- Once or twice a day (morning and lunchtime) administration is preferable.[46]

Visceral pain

Visceral pain can be:

- worse on taking a deep breath
- an excruciating pain – when an organ cannot swell to accommodate a tumour due to the presence of inflexible viscera containing the organ.

The most common example is liver pain due to metastases causing liver capsule stretch. Treatment is usually with morphine and steroids (dexamethasone 4–8 mg/day),[19] to reduce peri-tumour oedema. Palliative radiotherapy or chemotherapy may also be indicated.

Non-pharmacological management of pain

Transcutaneous electrical nerve stimulation (TENS)

The use of transcutaneous electrical nerve stimulation (TENS) machines has been found to be beneficial. Forty-seven per cent of patients report a 50% reduction in pain intensity after treatment.[47] TENS works by blocking the transmission of painful stimuli (referred to as the gate theory) by increasing activity in the large 'A' fibres, which block activity in the smaller pain fibres. There is a concomitant release of endorphins.

Pain receptive to TENS

- Back pain.
- Rib metastases or fractures.
- Sciatica.
- Post-herpetic neuralgia.
- Phantom limb pain.
- Musculoskeletal pain.
- Diabetic neuropathy.

Essential knowledge for TENS use

Dos:

- Read the manufacturer's instructions carefully before commencing treatment.
- TENS should be applied by an appropriately trained practitioner.
- Careful instruction and regular monitoring is necessary.
- Use pre-gelled adhesive pads.
- Settings vary according to the patient's pain.
- A starting frequency of 4–80 Hz, and pulse duration of 200 microseconds is a good baseline.
- Test the effectiveness of treatment for 20–30 minutes.
- Increase according to the response.
- > 12 hours a day may be required if the patient is not receiving any other analgesia.[48]

Do not:

- use the machine all the time
- place the electrodes
  - across the heart
  - on the side of the neck near the carotid arteries
  - on areas of broken or irradiated skin.

This could affect the heart rate, and/or cause electrode burns.

Checks and caution:

- If black rubber electrodes are used, check the pads regularly to ensure that there is sufficient electrode gel.
- Check and replace electrodes and electrode leads periodically.

Psychological approaches

Pain can be:

- physical
- spiritual
- emotional/psychological
- social.

This is referred to as *total pain*.[49]

Anxiety

Recognition that anxiety can increase the intensity of pain is essential and pivotal to any intervention.[7] The patient and family need continuous assessment and restructuring of care as identified. Some may benefit from counselling with regard to issues such as family problems, existential or spiritual needs in addition to analgesia.

Hope and coping strategies

Hope and coping strategies (e.g. distraction therapy, visualisation and imagery)[50] empower the individual, and enable better skills.

Relaxation and visualisation

Relaxation and visualisation can benefit the patient and family by:

- aiding sleep
- promoting management of stress and pain
- reducing anxiety and depression.[51]

Key tip 2.9

It may be appropriate to consult and or involve the community psychiatric nurse (CPN) during assessment, and for special guidance.

Pain and/or fear can cause tension, restlessness, poor concentration and agitation. Defined as a *state of freedom from both anxiety and skeletal muscle tension*, relaxation, for some patients and family, is helpful.[50] Simple breathing exercises can be helpful and explained during counselling.

Visualisation involves taking control of one's thoughts and distancing oneself from unpleasant situations.

Other pain management strategies

- Physiotherapy.
- Aromatherapy.
- Massage.
- Hypnotherapy.
- Osteopathy.
- Acupuncture.
- Spiritual healing.

Sometimes it is necessary to use a combination of techniques and/or relaxation in conjunction with other complementary therapies to provide an effective intervention. The decision on what is best is often trial and error and based on the patient's or family's experience and wishes.

Conclusion

Collaborative working and discussion with the interdisciplinary team and specialist palliative care team is important to achieve a common approach and optimise treatment outcome. Involving the interdisciplinary team throughout therapeutic interventions will ensure a team approach to the identified problems and will improve intervention and understanding of the nature of the pain and communication.

The key to effective pain management is continuous assessment and restructuring of interventions as directed by the patient or family who are experts in pain and their care.

The family role is pivotal to good quality care. They should never be excluded from pain assessment. It is extremely distressing to see one's wife/husband, partner, or child in chronic, unrelieved, pain. Therefore

- inclusion
- support
- guidance
- intervention
- opportunity

to discuss how the individual feels is imperative if therapeutic intervention is to be successful.

When assessing and planning intervention related to pain and its management, listening, and correct interpretation, is the primary tool. The correct use of the WHO analgesic ladder (*see* Figure 2.2) is useful in managing pain. Regular review is the best policy, using an appropriate validated pain-assessment tool where practicable.

Effective interventions mean *taking immediate action when pain is identified*. A prerequisite to good quality practice and intervention is awareness of new interventions and developments in drug and other therapies. The introduction of drugs such as transmucosal fentanyl lozenge and oxycodone liquid may give an additional boost to help manage rapid pain episodes. Early intervention with adjuvant analgesics maximises pain suppression.

It is important to continue supporting the individual even when interventions have not proved successful. Being present and alongside is a therapeutic intervention and encourages the therapeutic relationship.

Taking care of the patient and family is pivotal. However, of equal importance is the professional's need to take care of his- or herself. Being with someone in pain and deep distress is emotionally draining. Discussing one's feelings about the situation, and seeking support, within the context of regular supervision and good management is not a failing. It is good quality practice if our interventions on behalf of the patient and family are to be effective.

Self-assessment exercise 2.1
Time: 25 minutes

1 Your patient says the pain is burning and continuous in nature. What type of pain do you think this might indicate?
2 What drug treatment might be prescribed for nerve pain?
3 What are the *three steps* in the WHO analgesic ladder?
4 List three non-pharmacological treatments that may help to relieve pain.
5 Identify three non-verbal indicators that the patient may be in pain.
6 What are the common side effects of morphine?
7 When may fentanyl patches be indicated?

References

1 Twycross R. *Introducing Palliative Care*, 3rd edition. Oxford: Radcliffe Medical Press; 1999.
2 Murdoch J, Larsen D. Assessing pain in cognitively impaired older adults. *Nursing Standard*. 2004; 18(38): 33–39.
3 Abbey J, Piller N, Debellis A *et al*. The Abbey pain scale: a 1-minute numerical indicator for people with end-stage dementia. *Int J of Palliative Nursing*. 2004; 10(1): 6–13.
4 www.doloplus.com/versiongb/index.htm.
5 Doyle D, Hanks G, Cherney N *et al*., editors. *Oxford Textbook of Palliative Medicine*, 3rd edition. Oxford: Oxford University Press, p. 345.
6 Chandler A, Preece J, Lister S. Using heat therapy for pain management. *Nursing Standard*. 2002; 17(9): 40–42.
7 Stimmel B. *Pain and its Relief Without Addiction*. New York: Haworth Medical Press; 1997, p. 77.
8 Collin E, Poulain P, Piquard A *et al*. Is disease progression the major factor in morphine 'tolerance' in cancer pain treatment? *Pain*. 1993; 55: 319–326.
9 World Health Organization. *Cancer Pain Relief*, 2nd edition. Geneva: World Health Organization; 1996.
10 Twycross R, Wilcock A, Charlesworth S *et al*. *Palliative Care Formulary*, 2nd edition. Oxford: Radcliffe Medical Press; 2002.
11 Hanks G, Hoskin P, Aherne G *et al*. Explanation for potency of repeated oral doses of morphine? *The Lancet*. 1987; 1.2: 723–725.

12 Davis M, Walsh D. Rapid opioid titration in severe cancer pain. *European Journal of Palliative Care.* 2005; **12**(1): 11–14.

13 Hanks G, Doyle D. *Oxford Textbook of Palliative Care*, 2nd edition. Oxford: Oxford University Press; 1994.

14 Stoutz N, Bruera E, Suarez-Almazor M. Opioid rotation for toxicity reduction in terminal cancer individuals. *Journal of Pain and Symptom Management.* 1995; **10**(5): 378–384.

15 Kaiko R, Wallenstein M, Rogers R *et al*. Analgesic and mood effects of heroin and morphine in cancer patients with post operative pain. *New England Journal of Medicine.* 1981; **304**(25): 1501–1505.

16 Twycross R, Wilcock A, Charlesworth S *et al*. *Palliative Care Formulary*, 2nd edition. Oxford: Radcliffe Medical Press; 2002, pp. 186–187.

17 Ahmedzai S, Brooks D. Trans-dermal fentanyl versus sustained-release oral morphine in cancer pain: preference, efficacy, and quality of life. The TTS-fentanyl – comparative trial group. *J Pain and Symptom Management.* 1997; **13**(5): 254–261.

18 Ellershaw J, Kinder C, Aldridge J *et al*. Care of the dying: is pain control compromised or enhanced by continuation of the fentanyl trans-dermal patch in the dying phase? *Journal of Pain and Symptom Management.* 2002; **24**(4): 398–403.

19 Back I. *Pain in Palliative Medicine Handbook*, 3rd edition. Cardiff: BPM Books; 2001, p. 77.

20 Payne R, Chandler S, Einhaus M. Guidelines for the clinical use of trans-dermal fentanyl. *Anticancer Drugs.* 1995; Suppl. **6**(3):50–3.

21 Twycross R, Wilcock A. *Symptom Management in Advanced Cancer*, 3rd edition. Oxford: Radcliffe Medical Press; 2001, p. 381.

22 Hanks G, Nugent M, Higgs C *et al*. Oral transmucosal fentanyl citrate in the management of breakthrough pain in cancer: an open, multicentre, dose-titration and long term use study. *Palliative Medicine.* 2004; **18**: 698–704.

23 Flock P, Gibbs L, Sykes N. Diamorphine-metronidazole gel effective for treatment of painful infected leg ulcers. *Journal of Pain and Symptom Management.* 2000; **20**(6): 396–397.

24 Grocott P. Palliative management of fungating malignant wounds. *Journal of Community Nursing.* 2000; **14**(3): 31–40.

25 Naylor W. Assessment and management of pain in fungating wounds. *British Journal of Nursing.* 2001; Suppl. **10**(22): 33–56.

26 Zepetella G. Topical opioids for painful skin ulcers: do they work? *European Journal of Palliative Care.* 2004; **11**(3): 93–96.

27 Naylor W. Malignant wounds: aetiology and principles of management. *Nursing Standard.* 2002; **16**(52): 45–53.

28 Doyle D, Hanks G, Cherny N. *Oxford Textbook of Palliative Care*, 3rd edition. Oxford: Oxford University Press; 2003.

29 Mercadante S, Villari P, Ferrera P *et al*. Addition of a second opioid responses in cancer pain: preliminary data. *Support Cancer Care.* 2004; **12**: 762–766.

30 Kaye P. *A–Z of Hospice and Palliative Medicine*. Northampton: EPL Publications; 1992.

31 Toscani F, Piva L, Corli O *et al*. Ketorolac versus diclofenac sodium in cancer pain. *Arzeneim-forsch-drug-res.* 1994; **44**(4): 550–554.

32 Buckley M, Brogden R. Ketorolac: a review of its pharmacodynamic and pharmacokinetic properties and therapeutic potential. *Drugs.* 1990; **39**: 86–109.

33 Blackwell N, Bangham L, Hughes M *et al*. Subcutaneous keterolac – a new development in pain control. *Palliative Medicine.* 1993; 7: 63–65.

34 Micaela M, Brogen B, Brogen R. Keterolac – a review of its pharmacodynamic and pharmacokinetic properties, and therapeutic potential. *Drugs.* 1990; **39**(1): 86–109.

35 Myers K. What's new about NSAIDs? *Continuing Medical Education Bulletin Palliative Medicine.* 1999; 1(2): 31–33.

36 Johnson A. Use of bisphosphonates for the treatment of metastatic bone pain; a survey of palliative care physicians in the UK. *Palliative Medicine.* 2001; **15**: 141–147.

37 Ripamonti C, Fulfaro F, Ticozzi C *et al*. (1998) Role of pamidronate disodium in the treatment of metastatic bone disease. *Tumori.* 1998; **84**(4): 442–455.

38 Body J, Deal I, Bell R *et al*. Oral ibandronate improves bone pain and preserves quality of life in patients with skeletal metastases due to breast cancer. *Pain.* 2004; **111**(3): 306–312.

39 Twycross R. Wilcock A. *Pain Relief in Symptom Management in Advanced Cancer*, 3rd edition. Oxford: Radcliffe Medical Press; 2001, p. 27.

40 Osterland H, Beirne P. Complementary therapies. In: Ferrell B, Coyle N, editors. *Textbook of Palliative Nursing.* Oxford: Oxford University Press; 2001, pp. 374–375.

41 Nilsson S, Strang P, Ginman C *et al.* Palliation of bone pain in prostate cancer using chemotherapy and Strontium-89 – a randomized phase II study. *Journal of Pain and Symptom Management.* 2005; **29**(4) 352–357.

42 Kaye P. A–Z *Pocketbook of Symptom Control.* Northampton: EPL Publications; 2003, p. 112.

43 Rockafort J, Viquria J. Gabapentin as an analgesic: benefits and side-effects of using an anticonvulsant drug to combat neuropathic pain in a palliative care setting. *European Journal of Palliative Care.* 2001; **8**(2): 54–56.

44 Freynhagen R, Strojek K, Greising T *et al.* Efficacy of Pregabalin in neuropathic pain evaluated in a 12-week, randomised, double-blind, multicentre, placebo-controlled trial of flexible- and fixed-dose regimens. *Pain.* 2005; **115**(3): 254–263.

45 British Medical Association and the Royal Pharmaceutical Society of Great Britain. *British National Formulary: glucocorticoid therapy*, 49th edition. London: British Medical Association and the Royal Pharmaceutical Society of Great Britain; 2005, 6.3.2.

46 Edwards A, Gerrard G. The management of cerebral metastases. *European Journal of Palliative Care.* 1998; **5**(1): 7–11.

47 Johnson MI, Ashton CH, Thompson JW. An in-depth study of long term users of transcutaneous electrical nerve stimulation (TENS): implications for the use of TENS. *Pain.* 1991; **44**: 221–229.

48 Mitchell A, Kafai S. Patient education in TENS pain management. *Professional Nurse.* 1997; **12**(11): 804–807.

49 Saunders C. *Hospice and Palliative Care – an interdisciplinary approach.* London: Edward Arnold; 1990, p. 27.

50 Waugh L. Psychological aspects of cancer pain. *Professional Nurse.* 1988; **September**: 504–508.

51 McCaffrey M, Pasero C. *Pain: clinical manual*, 2nd edition. London: Mosby; 1999.

To learn more

Books

- Basford L. Complementary therapies. In: Basford L, Slevin O, editors. *Theory and Practice of Nursing: an integrated approach to caring*, 2nd edition. Cheltenham: Nelson Thornes; 2003, Chapter 31, pp. 569–596.
- Cooper J. Coping with death and bereavement. In: Basford L, Slevin O, editors. *Theory and Practice of Nursing: an integrated approach to caring*, 2nd edition. Cheltenham: Nelson Thorne; 2003, chapter 35, pp. 664–681.
- Doyle D, Hanks G, Cherny N *et al.*, editors. *Oxford Textbook of Palliative Medicine*, 3rd edition. Oxford: Oxford University Press; 2003.
- Regnard C, Tempest S. *A Guide To Symptom Relief In Advanced Disease*, 4th edition. Cheshire: Hochland and Hochland; 1998.
- Stimmel B. *Pain and its Relief Without Addiction.* New York: Haworth Medical Press; 1997.
- Twycross R, Wilcock A. *Symptom Management in Advanced Cancer*, 3rd edition. Oxford: Radcliffe Medical Press; 2001.
- Twycross R, Wilcock A, Charlesworth S *et al. Palliative Care Formulary*, 2nd edition. Oxford: Radcliffe Medical Press; 2002.
- Wall P. *Pain: the science of suffering.* London: Orion; 1999.

Websites

- British Pain Society: www.britishpainsociety.org/index.html.
- Behavioural pain-assessment scale and discussion for older patients with verbal communication disorders: www.doloplus.com/versiongb/index.htm.
- Discussion of pharmaceutical and other treatment of pain: www.palliativedrugs.com/pdi.html.
- Information on TENS machine settings: www.electrotherapy.org/electro/tens/tens.htm.
- Relaxation exercises: www.patient.co.uk/showdoc/27000363/.

Complementary chapters

See also Stepping into Palliative Care 1: relationships and responses

- Chapter 5: The psychological impact of serious illness
- Chapter 6: Hope and coping strategies
- Chapter 7: The therapeutic relationship
- Chapter 11: The value of teamwork
- Chapter 12: Stress issues in palliative care
- Chapter 13: Communication: the essence of good practice, management and leadership
- Chapter 16: Sexuality and palliative care

See also Stepping into Palliative Care 2: care and practice

- Chapter 1: Assessment in palliative care
- Chapter 4: Continuous subcutaneous infusion
- Chapter 8: Emergencies in palliative care
- Chapter 9: The last few days of life
- Chapter 12: Hearing the pain of the carer
- Chapter 13: Spirituality and palliative care
- Chapter 15: Complementary therapies: a therapeutic model for palliative care

Chapter 3

Symptom management: a framework

Susanna Hill

Introduction

Good management of physical symptoms is pivotal to the practice of compassionate palliative medicine. Symptoms are *'the problems a patient presents'*. Many factors affect how a symptom is presented. They include:

- the nature of the symptom
- the level of discomfort it causes
- what a patient understands about it
- what their fears are with regard to it
- what they think this means in terms of their illness
- any previous experiences they have had themselves or seen in family or friends of similar problems
- fear of possible outcomes if they report their symptoms in a certain way, e.g. medication or hospitalisation.

When assessing symptoms it is extremely important to pay attention not only to the occurrence of the symptom, i.e. timing, duration and severity, but to the meaning it has for the patient, i.e.:

- what effect it has on their daily living
- how distressing it is for them.[1]

In this way, the assessment should encompass the physical, social, psychological, emotional and spiritual dimensions of the problem for that person.

General principles

Patients with life-threatening conditions can present with many different symptoms. Although most of the data regarding these symptoms has been collected from observing patients with cancer, many patients in the end stages of life experience similar symptoms, regardless of the underlying pathology (*see* Box 3.1).

Box 3.1   Frequency of symptoms in patients with advanced cancer[2]

Pain	82%
Nausea and vomiting	59%
Dyspnoea	51%
Constipation	51%
Weakness	64%
Anorexia	64%
Depression	40%
Confusion	20%

It is rare for patients to present with a single symptom. The patient with multiple symptoms can be a daunting prospect for the professional.

This chapter does not replace the use of definitive texts on symptom management in palliative medicine. It aims to provide a *ten-step framework* to help you answer the question *'where do I start?'*. Case histories demonstrate how to use the framework to decide on the best method of treatment for the common symptoms you may encounter in patients receiving palliative care.

Ten-step symptom management framework

1 **What are the symptoms?**
   - Listen to the history and compile a list of symptoms.
   - Patients tend to under-report symptoms themselves when answering open questions.
   - Systematic questioning often reveals more problems.
2 **Prioritise symptoms to be dealt with first.**
   - This is the patient's priorities not yours, e.g.:
     - they may feel that their nausea is more difficult to cope with than their pain
     - you may feel their pain is the worst problem.
3 **Compile a list of potential causes of that symptom.**
   - Is the symptom due to:
     - the illness
     - the treatment
     - unrelated causes?
4 **Establish the probable cause of the symptom.**
   - Take a full history.
   - Explore the occurrence of the symptom, i.e.:
     - timing
     - frequency
     - duration
     - intensity.
   - Explore the meaning of the symptom.
   - Examine the patient appropriately.
   - Investigate as appropriate based on:
     - the history

    – examination

    – knowledge of the possible causes of the symptom

    – the patient's medical condition.

5 **Explore ideas, concerns and expectations (ICE).**
   - Find out what the patient knows and believes.
   - What are their ideas, concerns and expectations?

6 **Discuss the likely diagnosis.**
   - Use plain English not medical jargon.
   - 'Align' yourself with the patient.[3]
   - Incorporate their ideas and concerns in your explanation.
   - Provide enough information for a patient to be able to understand the problem and discuss treatment options with you.
   - Patients are more likely to agree to treatments if they:
     - understand why they may help
     - have had the opportunity to discuss options with you.

7 **Decide on the best treatment.**
   - Individualise the treatment based on:
     - your knowledge of the likely cause of the symptom
     - its meaning to the patient
     - the patient's treatment choice.
   - Consider both medical and non-medical options, e.g. metoclopramide vs acupuncture to treat nausea.

8 **Set realistic treatment goals – maintain hope.**[4]

9 **Assess the response –** *have you been*:
   - *successful?* – continue
   - *partially successful?* – optimise treatment and/or add another treatment
   - *unsuccessful?* – start again, reassess.

10 **Review! Review! Review!**
   - The condition of palliative care patients can deteriorate rapidly and the patient often needs constant reassessment.

Self-assessment exercise 3.1
Time: 20 minutes

- What are the ten steps in the symptom management framework?
- Categorise the causes of symptoms into three general groups.

Use the framework for the next patient you see with multiple symptoms:

- Did it help?

'I feel really sick': nausea and vomiting

Case scenario 3.1 (part 1)

June (56), an anxious lady, was diagnosed with carcinoma of the pancreas 9 months ago. Recently, June started vomiting large volumes of gastric contents, and complaining of a swollen abdomen and back pain. Current medication consists of morphine slow-release tablets (MST) 120 mg twice daily (bd) and metoclopramide 10 mg four times a day as necessary (qds prn).

Step 1: What are the symptoms?

- Nausea, vomiting, back pain and a distended abdomen.

Step 2: Prioritise symptoms

- Nausea.

For many patients constant nausea can be more distressing than intermittent vomits.

Step 3: List the potential causes

Due to the illness

- **GI tract:**
  - oral candida
  - gastric outflow obstruction from tumour or lymph nodes
  - squashed stomach
  - hepatic distension due to metastases
  - ascites
  - constipation
  - bowel obstruction.
- **Cerebral:**
  - taste/smell
  - fear/anxiety
  - cerebral secondaries.
- **Metabolic:**
  - hypercalcaemia
  - hyponatraemia
  - uraemia
  - tumour toxins.

Due to the treatment

- Drugs – opioids, NSAIDs (non-steroidal anti-inflammatory drugs), steroids.
- Chemotherapy.
- Radiotherapy.

Other causes

- Other GI tract problems, e.g. stomach or oesophagus.
- Peptic ulcer.
- Gall bladder disease.
- Reflux oesophagitis.
- Renal disease.
- Labyrinthitis.

Step 4: Establish the probable cause of the symptom

History

- What is the timing of the vomits?
- Is there a relationship to food, certain drugs, certain visitors?
- Is the vomiting associated with epigastric pain, e.g. peptic ulcer disease?
- Is it projectile or faeculent? More likely to have a high obstruction.
- Are her bowels working? Think of constipation or bowel obstruction.
- Is the associated nausea relieved by vomiting (more likely to have gastric stasis causing the problem) or does the nausea continue after vomiting (more likely to be due to 'toxins' such as drugs or metabolic disturbance).
- Are there any other symptoms such as vertigo?
- What does it mean to her? What is the effect on her daily life? Eating is a social event and a lot of family interaction occurs around mealtimes. Can she cook at all? What does she feel about losing weight? Does this mean progression of her disease? After all if you do not eat ... you die!
- Assessment tools such as visual analogue scales can be useful in initial assessment and ongoing monitoring of response to treatment.

Examination

- Look for masses, hepatomegaly, jaundice, epigastric tenderness, oral candida, ascites, constipation, etc.
- Assess abdominal distension – not always present in malignant bowel obstruction as multiple bowel loops are often involved.
- Abnormal bowel sounds – these can be very quiet on opioids.

Investigation

- This can include a full blood count, liver function tests, glucose, urea and electrolyte levels, calcium, abdominal X-ray and gastroscopy.

Case scenario 3.1 (part 2)

June's vomiting did not occur in relationship to anything in particular. It occurred at any time of day and consisted of large volume vomits. It was accompanied by almost constant nausea, which was only partially relieved by vomiting. She had a distended abdomen with shifting dullness, was slightly jaundiced and had a hard irregular palpable liver edge. She was clinically diagnosed as having ascites and hepatic metastases. Her basic blood indices and biochemistry were measured. They showed a mild anaemia with a haemoglobin level (Hb) of 9.5 g/dl and slightly raised bilirubin and alkaline phosphatase consistent with a mild obstructive jaundice.

The possible causes of June's nausea and vomiting were thought to be:

- gastric outflow obstruction
- squashed stomach syndrome
- ascites
- hepatic metastases
- drugs, i.e. opioids
- anxiety
- tumour toxins.

Steps 5 and 6: Explore ideas, concerns and expectations (ICE) and discuss the likely diagnosis

Case scenario 3.1 (part 3)

June admitted that she thought this constant vomiting must mean that her bowel was blocked and that her cancer must be growing. She did not think she was ever going to feel any better.

Step 7: Decide on the best treatment

It is important to identify the cause of nausea and vomiting, as treatment depends on the cause. The integrated vomiting centre in the hindbrain receives signals via afferent (incoming) nerves. These stimulate the vomiting centre which sends signals via the efferent (outgoing) nerves of the vagus to the stomach, upper gastrointestinal tract and diaphragm to cause vomiting. Each incoming signal from different areas of the body acts via a different chemical neurotransmitter on a receptor to trigger this response. Antiemetics are used to block the different receptors, the choice of drug depending on where the signal is coming from and which putative receptor is being stimulated (*see* Figure 3.1).

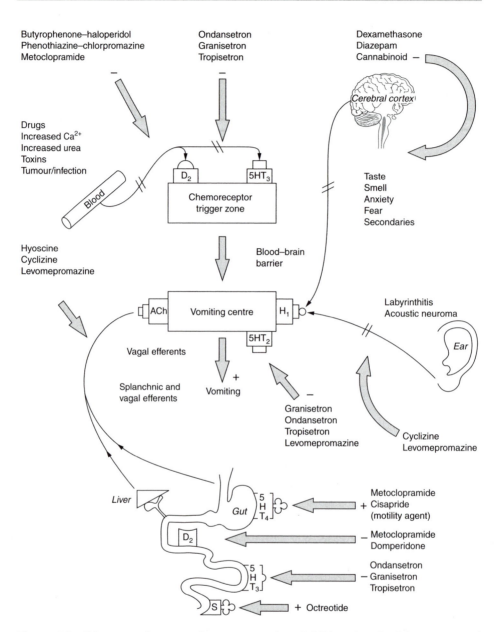

Figure 3.1 Triggers, pathways and neurotransmitter inhibitors involved in nausea and vomiting. Receptors: D_2, dopamine; S, somatostatin; AC, muscarinic cholinergic.

Key tip 3.1

Knowledge of the peripheral pathways and central neurotransmitters and receptors, which trigger nausea and vomiting, will enable you to choose the most effective antiemetic.

Options for treatment

- **General measures:**
  - minimise food and cooking smells
  - encourage snacks rather than large meals
  - arrange for someone else to do the cooking
  - encourage a calm environment.
- **Specific treatments** for conditions such as:
  - oral candida
  - peptic ulcer
  - gastritis
  - gallbladder disease
  - constipation
  - hypercalcaemia
  - drugs.

If no reversible cause for the nausea and vomiting can be found, consider the most likely cause. Decide which drug is likely to block the neurotransmitter being used by that afferent signal (*see* Figure 3.1).

If the nausea and vomiting partially respond to treatment, optimise the drug dose and, if still symptomatic, add or substitute a second drug.[5] If there is no response reassess the patient and see if there could be another cause for the persistent symptoms and change the treatment.

A stepwise approach to the management of nausea and vomiting can be adopted that is similar in many ways to the analgesic ladder used in pain management.[6,7]

Antiemetic ladder

- **Step 1:**
  - *Metoclopramide* – a prokinetic antiemetic which acts peripherally to stimulate peristalsis in the upper GI tract (for gastritis, gastric stasis and functional bowel obstruction). It also acts centrally on the dopamine receptors of the chemo-receptor trigger zone reducing most chemical effects of nausea and vomiting, e.g. drugs, uraemia, toxins and hypercalcaemia.
  - *Domperidone* – can also be used as a motility agent. Its prokinetic effect is exerted at the oesophago-gastric and gastroduodenal junctions – it does not cross the blood–brain barrier and so does not have any central effect.
- **Step 2:**
  - *Haloperidol* – acts principally on dopamine receptors in the chemoreceptor trigger zone for most chemical causes of nausea and vomiting (opioids, uraemia and hypercalcaemia).

and/or

  - *Cyclizine* – acts principally on histamine receptors in the vomiting centre (motion sickness, organic bowel obstruction and raised intracranial pressure together with dexamethasone).
- **Step 3:**
  - *Levomepromazine* – acts on dopamine, serotonin, acetylcholine and histamine receptors (organic bowel obstruction and when other antiemetics are unsatisfactory).

Other drugs to consider

- *Hyoscine butylbromide* – reduces bowel colic and gastric secretions.
- *Ondansetron/granisetron/tropisetron* – act on 5-HT3 receptors. Use when there is a massive release of 5-HT from enterochromaffin cells of the gut or platelets (chemotherapy, abdominal irradiation, bowel obstruction with distension, renal failure).
- *Olanzepine* – consider in bowel obstruction if levomepromazine is too sedating.[8]
- *Corticosteroids* – dexamethasone – as an adjuvant in bowel obstruction and at other times if all else fails. They possibly work by reducing the permeability of the blood–brain barrier and the CTZ (chemoreceptor trigger zone) to emetogenic substances. They may also reduce the amount of neurotransmitters in the hindbrain and GI tract.
- *Octreotide* – a somatostatin analogue that reduces gastric secretion and motility without antispasmodic effect. Use in bowel obstruction if hyoscine butylbromide is ineffective. Useful in large volume vomiting.
- *Ranitidine* – decreases gastric secretions as well as decreasing acidity. Proton pump inhibitors only affect acidity.
- *Nabilone* – a cannabinoid may be effective for intractable nausea and vomiting due to chemotherapy.[9]

Key tip 3.2

Antimuscarinic drugs such as cyclizine block the cholinergic pathways through which prokinetics work. Concurrent use blocks the action of metoclopramide and is best avoided.

Complementary treatments such as acupuncture, reflexology, aromatherapy and massage may all help. They may have a direct effect on nausea and vomiting but can also help to decrease anxiety and fear by helping the patient to relax. Behaviour/aversion therapy may help to reduce a learnt vomiting reflex in response to unpleasant stimuli such as chemotherapy or even the smell of the hospital!

Case scenario 3.1 (part 4)

It was decided to start June on a combination of haloperidol, to combat the nausea and vomiting due to opioids and tumour toxins, and cyclizine to help any symptoms due to ascites, hepatic disease and squashed stomach syndrome. These drugs were given subcutaneously via syringe driver to maximise effect and minimise discomfort.

Step 8: Set realistic treatment goals – maintain hope

Case scenario 3.1 (part 5)

The aim of treatment was to try and stop the nausea and perhaps reduce the vomiting to only once or twice a day. June felt that this would vastly improve her quality of life.

Step 9: Assess the response

Case scenario 3.1 (part 6)

Within 24 hours June felt much better. She had stopped feeling so nauseous and the frequency of her vomiting decreased to once or twice a day.

Step 10: Review! Review! Review!

Case scenario 3.1 (part 7)

June's condition deteriorated fairly rapidly. Her vomiting started to increase in frequency. She became far more anxious. To try and help with both these symptoms the haloperidol and cyclizine were replaced by levomepromazine in the syringe driver. She found the sedation this caused unpleasant but managed to cope with a reduced dose using massage as an adjunct to help her anxiety. It was only when certain family issues were addressed that she started to relax a bit more and become more accepting of her death. Her vomiting improved dramatically after this.

Self-assessment exercise 3.2
Time: 20 minutes

- List the common causes of nausea and vomiting.
- Draw a diagram to show how different stimuli act centrally to cause nausea and vomiting.
- Which neurotransmitter receptors are involved and where do various antiemetics work?
- What is the 'stepwise treatment' for nausea and vomiting?

'I can't breathe': breathlessness

> **Case scenario 3.2 (part 1)**
>
> Five years ago Lilly (72) underwent a right mastectomy for breast cancer. She subsequently developed a swelling in her right axilla and mild lymphoedema of her right hand. This was assumed to be due to secondary lymph node spread from her original tumour. She was treated initially with radiotherapy and started chemotherapy. However she only tolerated three cycles of treatment, as she felt extremely unwell with this. Six months later she presented in the GP surgery with increasing breathlessness and profound fatigue. She was extremely anxious about the change in her condition. Her only medication at the time was tamoxifen.

Step 1: What are the symptoms?

- Breathlessness, swelling of her right arm, anxiety and fatigue.

Step 2: Prioritise

- Breathlessness – this was preventing her from going out and enjoying her favourite hobby, ballroom dancing.

Step 3: List the possible causes (see Figure 3.2)

Due to the illness

- Lung metastases.
- Lymphangitis carcinomatosa.
- Pleural effusion.
- Ascites.
- Hepatomegaly.
- Pulmonary emboli.
- Superior vena cava obstruction (SVCO).
- Anaemia.
- Anorexia-cachexia, causing respiratory muscle weakness.

Due to the treatment

- Radiotherapy causing lung fibrosis.
- Chemotherapy, e.g. bleomycin.
- Other drugs – NSAID/aspirin causing bronchospasm and/or fluid retention, hormones predisposing to venous thrombosis and pulmonary embolism.

Other causes

- Infection.

- Asthma.
- COPD (chronic obstructive pulmonary disease).
- Pneumothorax.
- Fibrotic lung disease.
- Heart failure.
- Pericardial effusion.
- Neuromuscular weakness, e.g. motor neurone disease.
- Anaemia.
- Acidosis.
- Anxiety causing hyperventilation.

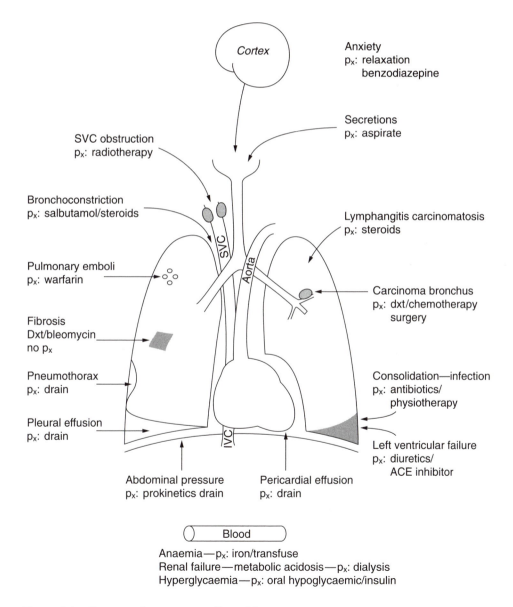

Figure 3.2   Causes and treatments of breathlessness.

Step 4: Establish the probable cause

History

- Previous chest problems, e.g. asthma, bronchitis?
- Is the breathlessness present at rest?
- Is the breathlessness present in bed, e.g. paroxysmal nocturnal dyspnoea with cardiac disease?
- Does anything make it worse, e.g. pollen in asthmatics?
- Does anything make it better?
- Does it respond to any medication?
- Has there been any haemoptysis suggestive of pulmonary embolism (PE), infection or metastases?
- Is there pain or palpitations – cardiac causes?

Examination

- Appearance – pink/blue – COPD, SVCO.
- Position of patient:
  - orthopnoea of heart failure patients (difficulty in breathing unless in an upright postion)
  - sitting forward leaning on elbows with COPD.
- Lymph nodes – metastases.
- Auscultation:
  - *wheeze* – space-occupying lesion, asthma
  - *crackles* – infection/fibrosis/lymphangitis carcinomatosa
  - *dullness* – effusion/consolidation.

Investigation

- More commonly – full blood count, chest X-ray (CXR), peak expiratory flow, spirometry, skin pulse oximetry, ECG (electrocardiogram), echocardiography and ventilation perfusion scan.
- MRI (magnetic resonance imaging) or CT (computerised tomography) scan of the chest, arterial oxygen saturation and Doppler scans of the leg veins may be helpful in specific cases.

Case scenario 3.2 (part 2)

Lilly's chest X-ray and full blood count were normal. Her spirometry showed a slightly restrictive pattern. This was thought to be due to mild COPD related to her previous smoking. A ventilation perfusion scan (VQ scan) was performed which showed small mismatched areas. A diagnosis of mild COPD and multiple pulmonary emboli was made. In this case, the predisposing factors for pulmonary emboli were malignant disease and tamoxifen.

Step 5: Explore ideas, concerns and expectations (ICE)

Case scenario 3.2 (part 3)

Lilly was very frightened and frustrated by her increasing breathlessness. Her worst fear was that she was eventually going to suffocate.

Step 6: Discuss the likely diagnosis

Establish the patient's understanding of the problem and discuss possible cause.

Step 7: Decide on the best treatment

The management of breathlessness relies on general measures relevant to all cases and more specific treatments related to specific causes of breathlessness.

General measures

- Sit upright.
- Reassure the patient – familiar faces help.
- Provide adequate ventilation – open window or use a fan to cool circulating air.
- Oxygen can help, but often more of a psychological support and use should perhaps be based on a low arterial blood concentration (*see* below).
- Morphine – linctus.
- Look at positioning of beds and chairs.
- Provide mobility aids.
- Provide commodes.
- Relaxation manoeuvres.
- Counselling and breathing retraining.[10]
- Complementary therapies including acupuncture and aromatherapy.

Specific measures

- Inhaled salbutamol, steroids , long-acting beta 2 agonists, Atrovent or Oxivent for asthma and COPD.
- Nebulised drugs if inhalation difficult.
- Radiotherapy for lung tumours causing haemoptysis or SVCO.
- Stenting for bronchial obstruction.
- Oxygen if the patient is hypoxic at rest [$SaO_2 < 90\%$ on skin pulse oximetry]. If $SaO_2 < 90\%$ after exertion offer oxygen for brief periods only to avoid over-dependence. Reduce the flow rate for those patients with COPD at risk of hypercapnia (increased amount of carbon dioxide in the blood).[11]
- Antibiotics for infection.
- Steroids and chemotherapy for lymphangitis carcinomatosa.
- Anticoagulation for pulmonary emboli.
- Diuretics and ACE (angiotensin-converting enzyme) inhibitors for cardiac failure.

- Iron or transfusion for anaemia.
- Benzodiazepines such as the shorter-acting lorazepam or buspirone for anxiety.

Case scenario 3.2 (part 4)

Lilly commenced on the bronchodilator salbutamol and atrovent to help her COPD. She did not respond to a trial of steroids and so these were not included in her management. She was also anticoagulated initially using low molecular weight heparin, followed by warfarin. Her tamoxifen was changed to anastrazole although it was appreciated that this is also thrombogenic.

Key tip 3.3

- Superior vena cava obstruction (SVCO) constitutes a relative emergency. Start treatment with 16 mg oral dexamethasone and low molecular weight heparin.
- Seek an urgent radiotherapy opinion.
- It is important to obtain a tissue diagnosis of cause before treatment is started if the diagnosis is unknown.

Step 8: Set realistic treatment goals

Maintain hope.

Case scenario 3.2 (part 5)

Lilly wanted to be able to ballroom dance again. She gradually accepted that this was not going to be possible and compromised on being able to get out to the tea dances, seeing her friends without the dancing!

Step 9: Assess the response

Case scenario 3.2 (part 6)

Although Lilly seemed to improve initially, her condition started to deteriorate again and her treatment seemed to make little difference to her increasing breathlessness.

Step 10: Review! Review! Review!

Case scenario 3.2 (part 7)

As she became increasingly breathless, Lilly became more and more distressed. She was given morphine linctus, 5 mg as needed, as she was opiate naive, and oxygen to use as necessary. She failed to improve and nebulised morphine was tried.[11] This did not help, so was stopped. General measures were implemented including trying to make sure she had company most of the time. She was offered relaxation tapes and psychological support to try and help her recognise and cope with the panic. A small dose of lorazepam was started – 0.5–1 mg three times a day as needed, as the risks of respiratory depression due to this were thought to be negligible compared to the benefits of reducing some of the anxiety.

Despite these efforts she continued to deteriorate. Her anxiety was a major problem. She never accepted that she might not get better. She was finally rushed into hospital acutely breathless and subsequently died from broncho-pneumonia.

The real reason for Lilly's continual deterioration was never established.

Self-assessment exercise 3.3
Time: 10 minutes

- What are the common causes of breathlessness?
- What non-pharmacological measures can be used to alleviate the symptoms of breathlessness?

'*I am so constipated*': constipation

Case scenario 3.3 (part 1)

Tommy (77), a retired farmer, has carcinoma of the prostate with bone secondaries. He has recently experienced increasing pain and has had his dose of MST increased to 130 mg twice daily (bd). His other medication includes diclofenac 50 mg three times a day (tds) for bone pain, and amitriptyline 75 mg once daily (od) for depression. He is complaining that his abdomen is distended and uncomfortable and that his bowels will not work.

Step 1: What are the symptoms?

- Pain, constipation and depression.

Step 2: Prioritise symptoms to be dealt with first

- Constipation is his greatest concern.

Step 3: Compile a list of potential causes of that symptom

Due to the illness

- Bowel obstruction.
- Hypercalcaemia.
- General debility.

Due to the treatment

- Drugs – opioids, antidepressants.

Other causes

- Poor diet.
- Lack of exercise.
- Poor fluid intake.
- Hypothyroidism.
- Electrolyte imbalance.

Step 4: Establish the probable cause of the symptom

History

- Is this true constipation, i.e. is the patient straining to pass hard stool?
- How long has this been a problem?
- When was the last time the patient managed to pass stools?
- Is he passing flatus?

Examination

- Does the patient have a distended abdomen?
- Is faeces palpable in the descending colon?
- Is the rectum full of hard stool?

Investigation

- Urea and electrolytes; calcium; thyroid function test.
- Abdominal X-ray – supine and erect.
  - If constipated the bowel will be full of faeces.
  - If obstructed there may be a large distended loop of bowel visible with multiple fluid levels seen on the erect film.

> **Case scenario 3.3 (part 2)**
>
> Tommy had a history consistent with constipation. On examination, he had a moderately distended abdomen with a rectum full of hard faecal pellets. The causes contributing to this were thought to be his medication (MST and amitriptyline), his depression and his general poor diet and debility.

Step 5: Explore ideas, concerns and expectations (ICE)

> **Case scenario 3.3 (part 3)**
>
> Tommy was anxious to get his bowels working again as he was sure this was the reason he felt so low and weak.

Step 6: Discuss the likely diagnosis

Establish the patient's understanding of the problem and discuss possible cause.

Step 7: Decide on the best treatment (see Box 3.2)

Specific measures

- Look at medication, e.g. change MST to less-constipating fentanyl,[9] change the antidepressant from a tricyclic to a less-constipating SSRI (selective serotonin reuptake inhibitor).
- Treat hypothyroidism if present.
- Treat hypercalcaemia if present.
- Increase dietary fibre and fluid intake.

General treatment

- Anticipate problems – start with treatment early, e.g. treat all patients on an opioid with a laxative.
- Titrate the dose and type of laxatives against the symptoms, e.g. are the stools soft but difficult to expel – use a stimulant. Are they hard and like rabbit pellets – use a softener.
- Aim to use both softeners/osmotic agent and a stimulant according to need.
- Fixed dose combinations help patient compliance but do not allow for flexibility in the ratio of softener to stimulant.
- In cases of faecal impaction, use enemas.

Box 3.2   Treatments for constipation

Bulking agents with high fibre content:

- fybogel
- normacol
- trifyba.

Softeners – osmotic agents drawing water into bowel:

- lactulose
- poloxamer
- docusate
- Movicol.

Stimulants:

- bisacodyl
- senna
- glycerine
- danthron.

Combination drugs:

- co-danthrusate (danthron and docusate)
- co-danthramer (danthron and poloxamer 1:8)
- co-danthramer forte (danthron and poloxamer 1:13).

Enemas:

- microlax
- phosphate.

Key tip 3.4

- Constipation can be of more concern to some patients than pain.
- Anticipate problems early – start treatment prophylactively.
- To treat effectively you often need a stool softener and stimulant.
- For bulking agents and osmotic laxatives to work effectively you need to increase fluid intake.

Case scenario 3.3 (part 4)

Tommy's diet was discussed and his fluid intake was increased. His MST was changed to a fentanyl patch 75 micrograms/hour and his amitriptyline was changed to sertraline. Microlax enemas were used initially to try and empty his rectum and relieve his discomfort. Co-danthramer forte 10 ml bd was introduced to soften and help expel his stools.

Step 8: Set realistic treatment goals

Maintain hope.

Case scenario 3.3 (part 5)

The aim of treatment was to be able to stop the use of enemas as soon as possible and for Tommy to pass a soft stool without straining every 2–3 days.

Step 9: Assess the response

Things improved initially.

Step 10: Review! Review! Review!

Case scenario 3.3 (part 6)

After 10 days Tommy developed faecal incontinence with watery diarrhoea. A rectal examination revealed a hard faecal mass impacted high in the rectum. He was diagnosed with constipation and overflow diarrhoea. He was given a phosphate enema and his dose of co-danthramer forte was increased to 20 ml twice daily (bd). His bowels settled into a more regular pattern but he remained depressed and in some pain.

Key tip 3.5

Diarrhoea can be due to constipation!

Self-assessment exercise 3.4
Time: 5 minutes

- Name the different laxatives used.
- How do the laxatives work?

'I can't go to the toilet': bowel obstruction

Case scenario 3.4 (part 1)

Emily (62) has disseminated ovarian carcinoma. She has locally invasive tumour and hepatic and lymph node secondaries. For 2 weeks, Emily has complained of increasing constipation and now complains of abdominal discomfort and nausea.

Step 1: What are the symptoms?

- Constipation, abdominal pain and nausea.

Step 2: Prioritise symptoms to be dealt with first

- Constipation.

Step 3: Compile a list of potential causes of that symptom

Due to the illness

- Tumour in the abdominal cavity.
- Functional paralytic obstruction.

Due to the treatment

- Adhesions following surgery.
- Ischaemic fibrosis post radiation.

Other causes

- Refer to surgical textbook for causes of bowel obstruction.

See Case scenario 3.3, Step 3, page 56, for causes of constipation.

Step 4: Establish the probable cause of the symptom

A patient may present with the classical symptoms of an acutely obstructed bowel, i.e. colicky abdominal pain, nausea and vomiting, and absolute constipation. However, in malignant disease, the presentation is often more insidious and variable. Patients may not be distended if there is multiple loop obstruction caused by autonomic nerve dysfunction. Bowel sounds may be quiet particularly if the patient is on opioids.[7]

History

- How long has the constipation been a problem?
- Is it absolute, i.e. no flatus or faeces?

- Is there any colicky pain?
- Is there any nausea or vomiting? This may be profuse if there is a high gastric outlet obstruction.

Examination

- Abdominal distension.
- Tympanitic bowel sounds.
- Abdominal mass.

Key tip 3.6

- In malignant bowel obstruction, the abdomen may be flat rather than distended if the obstruction is at multiple levels.
- Bowel sounds may be quiet rather than active if the patient is taking opioids.

Investigation

- Abdominal X-ray – erect/supine, to differentiate between constipation and bowel obstruction, or to see if there is a single large loop of bowel obstructed which might be amenable to surgery or stenting.
- Gastrograffin (*a contrast medium*) enema to determine the site of obstruction.

Case scenario 3.4 (part 2)

Emily had a 2-week history of increasing constipation, ending with absolute constipation over the last 5 days. She experienced nausea, vomiting and some mild colicky pains. Her abdomen was distended but there was no localised tenderness. Her bowel sounds were active, with an occasional tympanitic sound. Her rectum was empty.

A clinical diagnosis of bowel obstruction was made.

Steps 5 and 6: Explore ideas, concerns and expectations (ICE) and discuss the likely diagnosis

---

Case scenario 3.4 (part 3)

Emily understood that she had extensive disease. She did not want any interventive treatment. She agreed to palliative medical treatment of her bowel obstruction.

Step 7: Decide on the best treatment

Surgical management

This should be considered as an option for every patient. Up to a third of patients may have a non-malignant cause for their obstruction. Even when the obstruction is due to malignancy, many patients enjoy a considerable symptom-free period following palliative surgery. The option of inserting a stent to relieve an obstruction in the lower colon or rectum has increased the options for intervention.

Key tip 3.7

Always consider the option of surgery.

Medical management

- A small proportion of patients with a high gastric outlet obstruction may be more comfortable with nasogastric aspiration, but this should be the exception not the rule.
- In patients without colic who continue to pass flatus, a prokinetic drug is the drug of choice, e.g. metoclopramide.
- In patients who have or develop colic, prokinetic drugs should be stopped. An antisecretory, antispasmodic drug such as hyoscine butylbromide should be prescribed with an antiemetic such as cyclizine, haloperidol or levomepromazine.
- Bulk-forming and osmotic laxatives should be stopped. Try to keep the stool soft, e.g. use docusate.
- Morphine or diamorphine should be given for constant background cancer pain.
- Corticosteroids benefit some patients with inoperable intestinal obstruction. Because there may be a spontaneous resolution of obstruction in up to a third of patients, it is important not to treat too soon. If after 5–7 days symptoms have not improved with the above regime a trial of corticosteroid can be given.
- Octreotide can be considered if vomiting does not settle. This somatostatin analogue reduces secretions throughout the alimentary tract.
- Patients should be able to eat and drink as they choose.

Case scenario 3.4 (part 4)

Due to Emily's extensive disease and previous treatments medical management was agreed on. A syringe driver was set up containing diamorphine, hyoscine butylbromide and an antiemetic.

Step 8: Set realistic treatment goals

Maintain hope.

Case scenario 3.4 (part 5)

The aim was to reduce Emily's discomfort and enable her to eat small amounts of food.

Key tip 3.8

Most patients with bowel obstruction can be managed palliatively with medication, without the use of nasogastric aspiration.

Step 9: Assess the response

Case scenario 3.4 (part 6)

Emily's nausea settled quickly and she became pain free. She continued to vomit occasionally.

Step 10: Review! Review! Review!

Case scenario 3.4 (part 7)

After 7 days, Emily started to vomit again. She did not improve with a trial of dexamethasone and so a second syringe driver containing octreotide was set up. This helped to settle her symptoms.

Self-assessment exercise 3.5
Time: 5 minutes

- What are the treatment options for bowel obstruction?
- How should drugs be administered?
- Why?

'I can't do anything': fatigue/weakness

> **Case scenario 3.5 (part 1)**
>
> Margaret (50) has breast cancer. She has recently developed some lower thoracic back pain and has lost weight and become very tired and lethargic. She feels that her memory is deteriorating.

Step 1: What are the symptoms?

- Back pain, weight loss, pain, tiredness and loss of memory.

Step 2: Prioritise symptoms to be dealt with first

- Tiredness.

> **Key tip 3.9**
>
> Fatigue is nearly universal in patients with malignant disease. Therefore, it can be overlooked as a sign of serious but treatable disease.

Step 3: Compile a list of potential causes of that symptom

Due to the illness

- Tumour load.
- Anorexia/cachexia syndrome.
- Hypercalcaemia.
- Spinal cord compression.

Due to the treatment

- Drug accumulation, e.g. opioids, diazepam.
- Radiotherapy.
- Chemotherapy.
- Myopathy with steroids.

Other causes

- Anaemia.
- Infection.
- Anxiety/ depression.
- Insomnia.
- Anorexia.
- Cardiac failure.

- Respiratory failure.
- Metabolic disturbance, e.g. hyponatraemia, hypokalaemia.
- Thyroid disease.

Step 4: Establish the probable cause of the symptom

History

- Pay great attention to this – listen to what the patient says and to how it is said. This may well be your best clue to the diagnosis.
- What does the patient mean by tiredness/lethargy?
- When did it begin?
- Is the weakness localised or generalised?
- Does anything make it worse? Or better?

Examination

- Full physical examination including:
  - the nervous system
  - musculoskeletal system
  - mental state.

Investigation

- Directed by history and examination to include:
  - full blood count
  - urea and electrolytes
  - calcium
  - albumen
  - thyroid function tests
  - chest X-ray.

Beware of the following two conditions that can present with weakness:

1 *Hypercalcaemia* – presents with:
  - weakness
  - aching
  - nausea and vomiting
  - confusion
  - polyuria
  - constipation.

  It is usually due to the production of a parathormone-like protein by the tumour, a process that can be unrelated to the presence of bone metastases. A corrected calcium level of > 2.8 mmol/l is abnormal (check serum calcium/albumen to correct for low albumen).

2 *Spinal cord compression* – suspect this if the patient has any of the following:

  - back pain which is worse on lying
  - back pain which is worse on coughing or straining

- if there is a sensory change (usually one or two dermatomes below the level of compression), motor weakness or sphincter disturbance.

This is an emergency!

Key tip 3.10

Spinal cord compression is an emergency!

Case scenario 3.5 (part 2)

Margaret gave a history of generalised fatigue and overall weakness that had been slowly progressive until the last 2 weeks when it seemed to become much worse. Examination did not reveal anything of note. Her full blood count showed a mild anaemia of 9.8 g/dl. Her corrected calcium was raised at 3.5 mmol/l (normal range 2.2–2.6 mmol/l). A diagnosis of hypercalcaemia was confirmed.

Steps 5 and 6: Explore ideas, concerns and expectations (ICE) and discuss the likely diagnosis

---

Case scenario 3.5 (part 3)

Margaret had wondered if her symptoms were due to recurrent breast disease or if it was all due to her age. It was explained to her that her raised calcium level probably indicated further disease and that this would need to be investigated once her high calcium had been corrected.

Step 7: Decide on the best treatment

Specific measures

These are related to underlying pathology, e.g. antibiotics for infection, change opioid, transfuse if significant anaemia.

Hypercalcaemia:

- Decide whether to treat or not – is this a terminal event?
- New event, the patient's quality of life has been good, or it is a long time since the last episode – *treat*!
- Rehydrate the patient as necessary. Treat with bisphosphonates, IV pamidronate 60–90 mg in 500 ml 0.9% saline over 4 hours.

- Review the antitumour treatment. Monitor for recurrence – check the calcium level after 3 days if the symptoms have not improved significantly or every 2 weeks if the treatment appears to be successful.

Spinal cord compression:

- **Start treatment urgently.**
- Give dexamethasone, either 24 mg IV over 2 minutes if symptoms have been present for less than 1 week or 18 mg orally if deterioration has been slower.
- Arrange *immediately* to see an oncologist for a definitive diagnosis. This will usually require an MRI scan. Treatment is usually with radiotherapy. More rarely surgical decompression may be considered.

Non-specific measures

- Pacing and prioritising activities are important.
- If increased tumour load is suspected as a cause of weakness, consider giving dexamethasone 4 mg once daily (od). Stop after 1 week if there is no benefit. Maintain the drug at this level if it is beneficial, unless the patient has a prognosis of more than several months in which case the dose should be reduced.
- Medroxyprogesterone acetate 400 mg daily or megestrol 160 mg daily may also be tried to encourage weight gain and appetite.

Case scenario 3.5 (part 4)

Margaret was rehydrated with 3 litres of normal saline and then received a pamidronate infusion.

Step 8: Set realistic treatment goals

Maintain hope. Whether and how to treat the causes of fatigue and weakness must be weighed up carefully. Are these symptoms heralding terminal decline?

Case scenario 3.5 (part 5)

In Margaret's case, her deterioration had been rapid, her quality of life good and this was the first episode of hypercalcaemia. Treatment seemed totally justified.

Step 9: Assess the response

Case scenario 3.5 (part 6)

The aim of treatment for Margaret was to restore the ionised calcium level to normal and to improve the symptoms of fatigue, weakness and memory loss. Her calcium level dropped to below 2.8 mmol/l. She felt more energetic, stronger and her memory improved.

Step 10: Review! Review! Review!

Case scenario 3.5 (part 7)

Margaret was due to be fully assessed with a chest X-ray, CT scan and bone scan to try and locate the site of her recurrent tumour. While she was waiting for these investigations, she became aware of increasing pain in her back and some strange sensations in her feet. She had gone home for a few days and had to contact her community nurse as she developed some dribbling incontinence. Her GP happened to call in to see her that day and diagnosed an acute spinal cord compression. Dexamethasone 18 mg was given orally and Margaret was referred immediately to her local oncology centre. An MRI scan detected a compression of the spinal cord at the level of T12/L1 and radiotherapy was started within 12 hours of the diagnosis being made at home. Prompt action managed to save Margaret from paraplegia.

Key tip 3.11

Beware of the patient with:

- fatigue or weakness
- new back pain
- onset of urinary incontinence.

Self-assessment exercise 3.6
Time: 10 minutes

- List the common causes of weakness and fatigue.
- Name two important conditions that can present in this way.
- How do they present and how are they treated?

'He seems so muddled': confusion

Case scenario 3.6 (part 1)

David (50) has disseminated colon cancer with known hepatic secondaries. He is jaundiced and itchy. His wife, who is caring for him at home, contacts their GP in great distress as her husband has become very confused. She woke in the night and found him trying to get out of the front door to go to work.

Step 1: What are the symptoms?

- Confusion with disorientation in time and place, jaundice and itching.
- Consider his wife's distress.

Step 2: Prioritise symptoms to be dealt with first

- Confusion.

Step 3: Compile a list of potential causes of that symptom

Due to the illness

- Cerebral tumour (primary or secondary).
- Hypercalcaemia.
- Hepatic failure.

Due to the treatment

- Drugs, e.g. opioids, corticosteroids.

Other causes

- Biochemical abnormality, e.g. uraemia.
- Infection.
- Recent trauma.
- Alcohol or drug withdrawal.
- Cardiac failure.
- Respiratory failure.

Step 4: Establish the probable cause of the symptom

History

- Is it of recent onset? Suggests acute confusional state. Also suggested by a fluctuating course, disorganised thought, inattention, memory impairment and disorientation.
- A longer history, less symptom fluctuation and unchanged alertness suggests possible dementia.

Examination

- Relate to possible physical causes, e.g. chest examination.
- Perform a full neurological and mental health assessment.

Investigation

- According to physical findings, e.g. blood cultures, skull X-ray, MRI scan, etc.

Case scenario 3.6 (part 2)

David had become confused over a period of 3–4 days. His confusion seemed to vary throughout the day. He was particularly distressed at night when he became far more restless and wandered around the house.

His MST had been recently increased from 200 mg bd to 300 mg twice daily (bd), together with metoclopramide 10 mg qds prn, co-danthramer 10 ml bd and temazepam 20 mg at night. He had also been started on dexamethasone 4 mg daily 5 days earlier to help pain due to liver capsule stretching and his itching. Examination found him slightly jaundiced with a hard palpable liver edge. General physical examination was normal as was a full neurological examination including fundoscopy. Blood examination revealed a mild hypochromic anaemia. Hepatic function was impaired with a bilirubin level of 121 mmol/l (normal range < 17 mmol/l). An alkaline phosphatase level of 710 IU/l (normal range 20–130 IU/l) and lactate dehydrogenase (LDH) level of 2700 IU/l (normal range < 500 IU/l) were found. His calcium level, corrected for albumen level, was normal as were his urea and electrolytes.

David's confusion was diagnosed as being due to hepatic failure, possibly exacerbated by the introduction of dexamethasone and increase in dose of opioid.

Step 5 and 6: Explore ideas, concerns and expectations and discuss the likely diagnosis

---

Case scenario 3.6 (part 3)

Most of the discussion took place with David's wife, Mary. She understood that her husband was seriously ill. It was explained to her that his confusion was probably a sign of terminal disease, and that the aim of treatment would be to alleviate her husband's distress and anxiety.

Step 7: Decide on the best treatment

Specific measures

- Treat specific causes, e.g. antibiotics for infection, lower calcium levels if high.
- Alter any exacerbating drugs if possible, e.g. dexamethasone.

General measures

- Maintain familiar faces and surroundings.
- Maintain a light quiet environment.
- Keep to the same routine if possible.

Drugs

- Haloperidol 0.5–5 mg orally or subcutaneously stat, then tds. Then give hourly for two more doses if needed until settled. Most appropriate for the more confused, psychotic patient.
- Levomepromazine 25–50 mg subcutaneously stat if sedation is required.
- Midazolam 2–10 mg subcutaneously, repeated at 30-minute intervals as needed. Diazepam per-rectum (PR) can be given if the patient is acutely confused but not psychotic, and sedation is required.
- Other agents, e.g. promazine for agitation and risperidone for psychosis, can be considered.

Case scenario 3.6 (part 4)

General measures were looked at to help David. His dexamethasone was stopped and he was started on 5 mg haloperidol at night.

Step 8: Set realistic treatment goals

Maintain hope.

Case scenario 3.6 (part 5)

The aim was to try and improve the nights so that Mary could sleep. The hope was that David could stay at home. Night sitters were offered but Mary wanted to try and continue by herself at home.

Step 9: Assess the response

Case scenario 3.6 (part 6)

David's level of consciousness still fluctuated but his wandering at night improved and he seemed less distressed.

Step 10: Review! Review! Review!

Case scenario 3.6 (part 7)

Over the following days David became drowsier and weaker. His medication was changed from oral to subcutaneous administration via syringe driver. He subsequently died peacefully at home without further medication changes.

Self-assessment exercise 3.7
Time: 15 minutes

- How can one tell the difference between acute and chronic confusional states?
- What non-medical measures can be implemented to aid treatment?
- What pharmacological agents can be used to help treat confusional states?
- Which patients do they benefit?

Other common symptoms

What follows is not definitive but a brief discussion of other symptoms. It aims to cover a few practical salient points about each symptom and possible management.

Depression

A third of patients experience depression; therefore, how bad news is broken can affect the likelihood of developing depression.

Consider whether the patient is:

- quiet
- withdrawn
- tearful
- waking early
- anorexic
- feeling that life is worthless
- feeling suicidal.

An assessment of mood is often more helpful than physical symptoms as these may relate to the illness rather than depression, e.g. early morning waking may be due to pain rather than depression.

Treat with tricyclics or SSRIs. However, there is a need to be aware of side effects and risk of fatality in overdose with tricyclics. Consider cognitive behavioural therapy (CBT).

Urinary symptoms

Symptoms include:

- frequency
- urgency
- hesitancy
- retention
- spasms
- incontinence.

Treatments include:

- *infection* – antibiotic
- *urgency* – oxybutinin/imipramine
- *hesitancy* – indoramin/bethanacol
- *spasms* – consider oxybutinin/amitriptyline; monitor for infection, change catheter balloon size or catheter
- *consider* – specialist assessment and intervention.

Hiccups

Caused by:

- gastric distension
- diaphragmatic distension
- uraemia
- infection
- central nervous system (CNS) tumour.

Treatments include:

- rub the palate as far back as possible
- decrease gastric distension, e.g. with peppermint water, domperidone, meto-clopramide
- relax muscle, e.g. give baclofen, nifedipine, midazolam
- central inhibition, e.g. give haloperidol, chlorpromazine.

Pruritus

Caused by:

- uraemia
- bile salts
- skin disease
- drugs, e.g. opioids

- thyroid disease
- myeloma
- lymphoma
- polycythaemia rubra vera.

Treatments include:

- *simple measures* – moisturiser, cooler shorter baths, avoiding bath additives, e.g. bubble bath
- *drug treatments* – give antihistamines, dexamethasone, cholestyramine.

Terminal rattle

Caused by:

- secretions collecting in the oropharynx.

Treatment includes:

- try to reposition the patient
- explain the problem to the carers – they are often more distressed than the patient
- consider giving hyoscine hydrobromide or glycopyrronium
- it is better to treat early and try to prevent secretions accumulating
- treatment may need to be repeated or given subcutaneously
- if the patient is deeply unconscious, suction may be attempted.

Ascites

Often associated with peritoneal metastases.
  Treatment includes:

- treat causing discomfort, vomiting or dyspnoea
- diuretics, e.g. try frusemide or spironalactone, but paracentesis is usually necessary
- if the prognosis is extended, consider a shunt which drains the ascitic fluid back into the venous system.

Flushes/sweats

Caused by:

- hormonal manipulation
- chemotherapy
- radiotherapy
- tumour – usually with hepatic secondaries
- infection
- myeloma
- drugs, e.g. opioids.

Treatment includes:

- treat specific causes
- if pyrexic with sweats – give NSAIDs

- if no pyrexia consider giving propantheline
- acupuncture can relieve sweats due to hormonal imbalance.

Conclusion

The patient's condition constantly changes. Just as one problem seems to improve, another appears. For patients in the terminal phase of their illness such change can occur with frightening rapidity. Be aware of this. At every patient contact, remember to '**review, review, review!**'.

Patients are individuals. They have their own healthcare beliefs, fears and ideas. Listen to the individual. Give time – s/he has so much to tell us!

References

1 Aranda S. A framework for symptom assessment. In: O'Connor M, Aranda S, editors. *Palliative Care Nursing: a guide to practice*, 2nd edition. Oxford: Radcliffe Publishing; 2003.
2 Donnelly S, Walsh D. The symptoms of advanced cancer. *Semin Oncol.* 1995; **22**: 67–72.
3 Buckman R. *How to Break Bad News*. London: Pan; 1994.
4 Links M, Kramer J. Breaking bad news: realistic vs unrealistic hopes. *Support Cancer Care.* 1994; **2**: 91–93.
5 Lichter I. Which antiemetic? *J Palliative Care.* 1993; **9**: 42–50.
6 Twycross R, Back I. Nausea and vomiting in advanced cancer. *Eur J of Palliative Care.* 1998; **5**: 39–44.
7 Twycross R. Anorexia, cachexia, nausea and vomiting. *Medicine.* 2004; **32**(4): 9–13.
8 Jackson WC, Tavernier L. Olanzepine for intractable nausea in palliative care patients. *J Palliative Medicine.* 2003; **6**(2): 251–255.
9 Twycross R, Wilcock A, Charlesworth S *et al. Palliative Care Formulary*, 2nd edition. Oxford: Radcliffe Medical Press; 2002.
10 Breslin E. Breathing retraining in chronic obstructive pulmonary disease. *Journal of Cardiopulmonary Rehabilitation.* 1995; **15**: 25–33.
11 Ahmedzai S, Shrivastav SP. Breathlessness. *Medicine.* 2004; **32**(4): 14–16.

To learn more

Books

- Back IN. *Palliative Medicine Handbook*, 3rd edition. Cardiff: BPM Books; 2001.
- Doyle D, Hanks G, Cherny N. *Oxford Textbook of Palliative Medicine*. Oxford: Oxford University Press; 2004.
- Fallon M, O'Neill B. *ABC of Palliative Care*. London: British Medical Journal Books; 1998.
- Faull C, Woof R. *Palliative Care*. Oxford: Oxford University Press; 2002.
- Kaye P. *Decision Making in Palliative Care*. Northampton: EPL Publications; 1999.
- Kaye P. *A–Z Pocketbook of Symptom Control*. Northampton: EPL Publications; 1994.
- Thomas K. *Caring for the Dying at Home*. Oxford: Radcliffe Medical Press; 2003.
- Twycross R, Wilcock A. *Symptom Management in Advanced Cancer*. Oxford: Radcliffe Medical Press; 2001.
- Twycross R, Wilcock A, Charlesworth S *et al. Palliative Care Formulary*, 2nd edition. Oxford: Radcliffe Medical Press; 2002.

Website

- CLIP 15-minute online tutorials: www.helpthehospices.org.uk.

Complementary chapters

See also Stepping into Palliative Care 1: relationships and responses

- Chapter 3: The cancer journey
- Chapter 4: The experience of illness
- Chapter 5: The psychological impact of serious illness
- Chapter 6: Hope and coping strategies
- Chapter 8: Gold Standard Framework: a programme for community palliative care
- Chapter 9: Integrated care pathways
- Chapter 10: Terminal restlessness
- Chapter 14: Ethical dilemmas

See also Stepping into Palliative Care 2: care and practice

- Chapter 1: Assessment in palliative care
- Chapter 2: Introduction to pain management
- Chapter 4: Continuous subcutaneous infusion
- Chapter 8: Emergencies in palliative care

Continuous subcutaneous infusion

Andrew Dickman

Pre-reading exercise 4.1
Time: 10 minutes

- Consider the last time one of your patients had a syringe driver.
- Reflect on your knowledge at that time.
- Why was the syringe driver used?

What is a syringe driver?

A syringe driver is a battery-powered device that is used to deliver a continuous subcutaneous infusion. There are several devices currently available (*see* Figure 4.1). The devices are simple to use and deliver the contents of a syringe accurately over a predetermined time period.

Key tip 4.1

- Do *not* place mobile phones near syringe drivers.
- All devices described in this chapter are designed to safely stop should high levels of electromagnetic interference be encountered.

What syringe drivers are available?

At present, four syringe drivers may be encountered (*see* Figure 4.1). The Graseby MS26 and MS16A syringe drivers, together with the Micrel MP Daily, are discussed below. Although available, the Micrel MP mlh is not particularly suited to the palliative care setting and will not be discussed further. *In any setting, the use of a single type of syringe driver is strongly recommended in order to avoid potentially harmful mistakes.* In situations where this is not possible, procedures should be in place to ensure staff are fully trained and are confident with the different types of device. See Table 4.1 for a summary of the properties of the three syringe drivers.

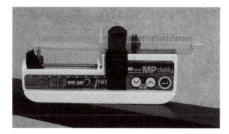

Micrel MP daily

- Size 165 mm × 40 mm × 23 mm
- Weight 190 g
- Uses 6 × alkaline AAA 1.5V batteries
- Battery life of approximately 50 infusions
- Wide variety of size and brand of syringe

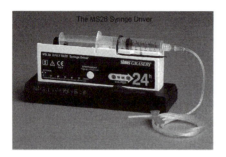

Graseby MS26

- Size 165 mm × 53 mm × 23 mm
- Weight 180 g
- Uses 1 × alkaline PP3 9V battery
- Battery life of approximately 50 infusions
- Wide variety of size and brand of syringe

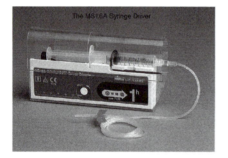

Graseby MS16A

- Size 165 mm × 53 mm × 23 mm
- Weight 180 g
- Uses 1 × alkaline PP3 9V battery
- Battery life of approximately 50 infusions
- Wide variety of size and brand of syringe

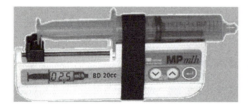

Micrel MP mlh

- Size 165 mm × 40 mm × 23 mm
- Weight 190 g
- Uses 6 × alkaline AAA 1.5V batteries
- Battery life of approximately 50 infusions
- Currently accepts only 20 ml BD Plastipak

Figure 4.1 The four available syringe drivers. (Adapted, with kind permission, from Dickman A, Schneider J, Varga J. *The Syringe Driver. Continuous subcutaneous infusions in palliative care.* Oxford: Oxford University Press; 2005.)

Table 4.1 Some properties of syringe drivers

Device	Rate of delivery	Maximum length of delivery	Syringe brand	Syringe size	Battery life
MP Daily	mm per 24 hours	60 mm	Any brand	Max 60 ml*	50 infusions
MS26	mm per 24 hours	60 mm	Any brand	Usual max 35 ml	50 infusions
MS16A	mm per hour	60 mm	Any brand	Usual max 35 ml	50 infusions

* Requires adjustment by manufacturer to allow this size of syringe to be attached.

MS26 and MS16A

- Very simple to use.
- Errors with identification have occurred and continue to occur.
- Poor safety features with only simple alarms.
- The syringe can easily become unattached.
- The infusion rate can be altered during the course of the infusion.
- The MS26 has a boost facility which must not be used for the following reasons:
    - The bolus dose of any analgesic delivered by the boost is far below the dose required for breakthrough pain. Each press of the boost button moves the plunger by 0.23 mm. *For a syringe containing 60 mg diamorphine, with a length of 18 mm, 0.23 mm would equate to 0.76 mg; the correct breakthrough dose should be 10 mg.*
    - The delivery of a boost dose is painful.
    - There will invariably be other medication in the syringe and bolus doses of these should not be given.
    - The infusion time will be reduced, giving rise to problems with renewal.
    - If the boost button is continually depressed, the MS26 will deliver a maximum of eight bolus doses before alarming, although the infusion will continue. However, if the boost button is released and depressed again, the process will be repeated, with the potential for the whole syringe contents to be delivered in a short space of time.
- Both have a delivery rate determined by mm of syringe-plunger travel.
    - MS26 delivers at a rate of mm per day
    - MS16A delivers at a rate of mm per hour.
    The *length of liquid* in the syringe, not volume, is important when setting the rate of delivery. This allows for flexibility and permits the user to attach a variety of sizes and brand of syringe.
- There is a maximum syringe-barrel length of 60 mm per infusion with these syringe drivers (i.e. the maximum distance that the syringe plunger can be extended and still fit on the syringe driver is 60 mm). A 20 ml syringe, for example, may contain a volume of 17 ml with a barrel length of 60 mm.

MP Daily

- Similar to the MS26, but more sophisticated (although more complicated to use).

- The delivery rate is determined by mm of syringe-plunger travel; it delivers at a rate of mm per day.
- There is a maximum syringe-barrel length of 60 mm per infusion (i.e. the maximum distance that the syringe plunger can be extended and still fit on the syringe driver is 60 mm). A 20 ml syringe, for example, may contain a volume of 17 ml with a barrel length of 60 mm.
- The MP Daily has improved safety features compared to the MS26:
  - No boost facility.
  - More secure syringe attachment.
  - The infusion rate cannot be altered once the infusion has started (unless the device is switched off and on again).
  - The infusion rate can be fixed, zoned or limited, reducing the risk of incorrect rate setting.
  - Variety of alarms that serve to improve the safety of the device include: occlusion alarm, low battery (one infusion remaining), depleted battery, end of plunger travel (i.e. syringe empty), system malfunction.

Why use a syringe driver?

> **Self-assessment exercise 4.1**
> **Time: 10 minutes**
>
> - Why is a syringe driver used for the administration of medication?
> - Make a list and compare your answers to those below.

Contrary to popular misconceptions, a syringe driver does not necessarily provide superior analgesia, nor does it signal impending death. A syringe driver should not be used as the 'fourth step' of the World Health Organization's analgesic ladder and intractable pain is *not* an indication. Patients occasionally appear to respond better to injections of diamorphine (or morphine) than they do to oral morphine. This can be explained by the poor absorption of morphine from the bowel. Rather than indicate that a syringe driver is needed, this may signal that an increase in oral dose of morphine is necessary, or perhaps a change to oral oxycodone is warranted. There are several reasons why a syringe driver may be used to administer medication:

- nausea and/or vomiting
- dysphagia
- severe weakness
- bowel obstruction
- diarrhoea
- unconsciousness
- patient request.

What are the advantages of using a syringe driver?

- Smooth medication delivery, increasing the patient's comfort by avoiding high and low blood levels.
- No need for repeated injections.
- Once-daily set-up generally required.
- Many symptoms can be managed by the use of a combination of medications.
- Patient's independence is maintained because the devices are small, light and easily portable.

What are the disadvantages of using a syringe driver?

- Associated with dying, or as the last resort.
- Site reactions are possible (although the risk can be minimised – see below).
- No flexibility with once-daily set-up.
- Training of staff must be maintained, particularly if more than one syringe driver is in use.
- Some patients dislike the idea of being attached to a device.

What diluent should be used?

The choice of diluent is still open to debate. The current situation is to dilute with Water for Injections, although for certain drugs, saline 0.9% may be better (e.g. levomepromazine). *Both diluents can be used for virtually all mixtures* (but note the exceptions for saline 0.9% below), although stability information is lacking.

Water for Injections tends to be more irritant, so certain mixtures are better diluted with saline 0.9%. It is therefore a plausible suggestion that for reasons of improved site tolerability and simplification, all mixtures should be diluted with sodium chloride 0.9% *except* for the following, where Water for Injections should be used:

- mixtures containing cyclizine (crystals form with saline 0.9%)
- mixtures containing diamorphine > 40 mg/ml; e.g. for a 20 ml syringe, where 60 mm = 17 ml, a concentration of 680 mg/17 ml = 40 mg/ml (crystals form with saline 0.9%).

How do I set up the syringe driver?

> **Key tip 4.2**
>
> - A 20 ml syringe is the *recommended minimum*.
> - Diluting the mixture to the maximum volume will reduce both the risks of adverse site reactions and incompatibility.
> - The amount of drug lost in the infusion set will be reduced, so the issue of priming the line becomes less important (*see* Box 4.1).

For all three syringe drivers:

- Ensure the patient and carer(s) are informed as to:
  - what a syringe driver is
  - why it is being used
  - how it works.
  Ensure they understand the advantages and possible disadvantages of using a syringe driver.
- Decide on a suitable site for infusion. Avoid damaged areas of skin, skin that has recently undergone irradiation, and oedematous areas. In general, for ambulatory patients, the chest or abdominal wall are suitable sites; for bedbound patients, the upper aspect of the arms can also be used; for distressed patients, siting around the scapula may be helpful in preventing the accidental displacement of the needle; in difficult situations, the thigh can be used.

MS26 and MS16A

The following steps should be followed when setting up the MS26 or MS16A syringe driver:

1 Fill the syringe with medication and dilute mixture to:
  a a maximum length of 60 mm for the MS26 and
  b a *fixed* length of 48 mm for the MS16A.
  Use the millimetre scale on the syringe driver for reference.
2 Prime the infusion line, if required (*see* Box 4.1).
3 Measure the length of barrel against the millimetre scale on the syringe driver.
4 Set the delivery rate by adjusting the screws on the front of the device. The rate is derived by dividing the length of the liquid by the required infusion time.

Rate setting for MS26:

$$\frac{\text{length of liquid (mm)}}{\text{infusion time (day)}} = \text{rate of infusion (mm/day)}$$

Rate setting for MS16A:

$$\frac{\text{length of liquid (mm)}}{\text{infusion time (hour)}} = \text{rate of infusion (mm/hour)}$$

Examples are shown below. Note the infusion time for the:

- *MS26 is calculated in days (per 24 hours)*
- *MS16A is calculated in hours.*

Driver	Length of barrel	Duration of infusion	Rate of infusion
MS26	60 mm (variable)	24 hours (1 day)	60 mm/24 hours
	48 mm (fixed)	12 hours (0.5 days)	96 mm/24 hours
MS16A	48 mm (fixed)	24 hours	2 mm/hour
	48 mm (fixed)	12 hours	4 mm/hour

5 Attach the syringe to the syringe driver, ensuring it is held tightly within the driver and the plunger of the syringe fits firmly within actuator.

6 Attach the giving set to the syringe.

7 Site the needle and secure the tubing with an appropriate dressing.

8 Insert the battery and an audible alarm sounds. This is the noise the device makes when:

- the infusion has ended
- the line is blocked
- the start/boost button is depressed for 10 seconds (MS26)
- the start/test button is held down for 5 seconds (MS16A).

9 Press the start button to silence the alarm and to activate the driver. If the light on the front of the driver does not flash (MS26 – every 25 seconds; MS16A – every second), replace the battery. *Providing the battery flashes at the start of the infusion, the syringe driver will be able to deliver an infusion for a further 24 hours.* If the light stops flashing during an infusion, replace during the next set-up procedure.

10 The syringe driver and syringe contents should be regularly checked.

11 An alkaline 9V battery, as recommended by Graseby, should be able to deliver 50 daily infusions.

Micrel MP Daily

The following steps should be followed when setting up the MP Daily syringe driver:

1 Turn the device on by depressing both chevron buttons until the device beeps.

2 Fill the syringe with medication and dilute mixture, up to a maximum length of 60 mm. Use the millimetre scale on the driver for reference.

3 Prime the infusion line, if required, before measuring and attaching the syringe (*see* Box 4.1).

4 Measure length of barrel against the millimetre scale on the syringe driver.

5 Attach the syringe to the device, ensuring a firm fixing.

Box 4.1   Priming the line. (Adapted, with kind permission, from Dickman A, Schneider J, Varga J. *The Syringe Driver. Continuous subcutaneous infusions in palliative care*. Oxford: Oxford University Press; 2005.)

If the syringe is measured *before* priming the infusion line, the syringe driver will run through early:

$$\frac{\text{Volume of infusion line}}{\text{Total volume in syringe}} \times \text{infusion time (hrs)}$$

The longer the infusion line, the earlier the infusion will end. For example, consider 1ml and 2 ml infusion lines and a 10 ml syringe volume over a 24-hour period:

$$\frac{1 \text{ ml}}{10 \text{ ml}} \times 24 \text{ hours} = 2 \text{ hours } 24 \text{ mins early}$$

$$\frac{2 \text{ ml}}{10 \text{ ml}} \times 24 \text{ hours} = 4 \text{ hours } 48 \text{ mins early}$$

If the syringe is measured *after* priming, the patient will not receive the prescribed dose:

$$\frac{\text{Volume of infusion line}}{\text{Total volume in syringe}} \times 100\%$$

Again, the longer the line, the greater the amount of drug the patient does not receive. For example, consider 1 ml and 2 ml lines and a 10 ml syringe volume over a 24-hour period:

$$\frac{1 \text{ ml}}{10 \text{ ml}} \times 100\% = 10\% \text{ of dose not received}$$

$$\frac{2 \text{ ml}}{10 \text{ ml}} \times 100\% = 20\% \text{ of dose not received}$$

Increasing the volume within the syringe reduces the impact of priming the line whether performed before or after the length of liquid has been measured:

$$\frac{1 \text{ ml}}{20 \text{ ml}} \times 24 \text{ ml} = 1 \text{ hour } 12 \text{ mins early}$$

$$\frac{1 \text{ ml}}{20 \text{ ml}} \times 100\% = 5\% \text{ of dose not received}$$

6 Set the delivery rate. This is derived by dividing the length of the liquid by the required infusion time. As with the MS26, the infusion time for the MP Daily is calculated in *days*.

$$\frac{\text{length of liquid (mm)}}{\text{infusion time (day)}} = \text{rate of infusion (mm/day)}$$

The rate is set by pressing the two chevron buttons to increase or decrease the value.

7 Start the infusion by holding the 'enter' button for 3 seconds. Two flashing horizontal bars on the display confirm the infusion is running. Unlike the MS26 and MS16A, the rate cannot be altered once the infusion has started. If the depleted battery alarm warning occurs, the MP Daily will continue to deliver the infusion for up to 24 hours; the batteries should be replaced during the next set-up.
8 The syringe driver and syringe contents should be regularly monitored.
9 The six alkaline AAA batteries that the MP Daily uses should last for 50 infusions.

What drugs can be used?

Self-assessment exercise 4.2
Time: 10 minutes

- List the commonly used syringe driver drugs.
- Compare your list with Table 4.2.

The list of drugs that can be delivered by a continuous subcutaneous infusion is forever increasing. However, Table 4.2 shows a list of drugs commonly used.

Site reactions

Occasionally, a patient develops a local skin reaction at the site of a continuous subcutaneous infusion. There are several causes, which include drugs and nickel allergy. The risk of developing a site reaction can be reduced by:

- rotating the site at least every 72 hours
- using sodium chloride 0.9% as the diluent (except for mixtures containing cyclizine, or where doses of diamorphine exceed 40 mg/ml)
- diluting the mixture as much as possible (especially if high doses of diamorphine are used)
- using a 12-hourly instead of 24-hourly infusion (allows for greater dilution)
- changing the cannula to one coated with Teflon
- changing the choice of drug(s) – cyclizine, levomepromazine and increasing doses of diamorphine are known to be the main drugs implicated in site reactions

Table 4.2 List of drugs that can be administered via a syringe driver

Drug	Indication(s)	Usual 24-hour starting dose	Usual stat dose	Common unwanted effects	Additional information
Diamorphine	Severe pain	5–10 mg	One-sixth total daily dose	Usual opioid adverse effects such as nausea, constipation, sedation and confusion	Diamorphine preferred choice in UK. Oxycodone suitable alternative. Morphine is available in most countries
Morphine		10–15 mg			
Oxycodone		10–15 mg			
Ketorolac	Bone pain	60 mg	30 mg	Gastro-duodenal toxicity	Must consider gastroprotection, e.g. lansoprazole
Cyclizine	Nausea/ vomiting	100–150 mg	50 mg	Mainly sedation	Useful for most cases. Must not be used in patient with severe heart failure
Haloperidol		5–10 mg	1.5–5 mg	Extrapyramidal effects	Useful for drug-induced nausea/ vomiting. Is used for agitation at higher doses
Levomepromazine		6.25–25 mg	6.25–12.5 mg	Sedation	Excellent antiemetic useful in refractory cases. *Not used first-line* due to sedation. Is used for agitation at higher doses
Metoclopramide		30–60 mg	10 mg	Bowel colic; extrapyramidal effects	Useful for gastric stasis. Must not be used if bowel obstruction suspected
Ondansetron		8–16 mg	4 mg	Headache, constipation	Useful for chemotherapy/ radiotherapy. Occasionally added to treatment of bowel obstruction
Octreotide	Bowel obstruction, carcinoid	300–600 micrograms	100 micrograms	May affect diabetic control	Used to treat symptoms of carcinoid. If giving stat injections, warm ampoule to room temperature to reduce pain before administration

Table 4.2 Continued

Midazolam	a Sedation/ anxiolytic b Anti- convulsant	a 10 mg b 20 mg	5–10 mg	Generally well tolerated	Higher dosages for anticonvulsant effect, especially if patient previously taking oral anticonvulsants
Glycopyrronium	Bowel obstruction, bowel colic, terminal secretions	600 micrograms	200 micrograms	Dry mouth, constipation	Glycopyrronium tends to be the anticholinergic drug of choice. All three are useful at reducing the volume of vomit. None has been shown to be superior for terminal secretions
Hyoscine butylbromide		60 mg	10–20 mg		
Hyoscine hydrobromide		1.2 mg	400 micrograms	As above, but also causes drowsiness and blurred vision	Rarely used now due to adoption of other, better tolerated drugs. Occasionally used as antiemetic

- adding low-dose dexamethasone (1 mg) to the syringe: this is a last resort – there are anecdotal reports of success, but the stability of the resultant mixture cannot be assured.

Conclusion

Syringe drivers provide an excellent safe and effective method of delivering a variety of medications. Contrary to popular belief, a syringe driver does not necessarily provide better analgesia, nor does it mean the patient's death is impending. Personnel involved in setting up syringe drivers should be fully trained and it is recommended that *regular education sessions* are held.

Self-assessment exercise 4.3
Time: 30 minutes

1 What is a syringe driver?
2 List the driver(s) that can be set at an hourly rate.
3 List the driver(s) that can be set at a daily rate.
4 Is increasing pain an indication for starting a syringe driver?
5 Name three areas of the body that are suitable infusion sites.
6 Should the boost button of the MS26 be used?

(*See* answers on page 88.)

To learn more

- Dickman A, Schneider J, Varga J. *The Syringe Driver. Continuous subcutaneous infusions in palliative care*, 2nd edition. Oxford: Oxford University Press; 2005.
- Twycross R, Wilcock A, Charlesworth S *et al*. *The Palliative Care Formulary*, 2nd edition. Oxford: Radcliffe Medical Press; 2002.
- Watson M, Lucas C, Hoy A, Back I. *Oxford Handbook of Palliative Care*. Oxford: Oxford University Press; 2005.

Answers to Self-assessment exercise 4.3

1 A battery-powered device that is used to deliver a continuous sub-cutaneous infusion.

2 MS16A, MP mlh.

3 MS26, MP Daily.

4 No, increasing pain is not an indication.

5 Chest, abdomen, arm, thigh, back.

6 The boost button on the MS26 must *never* be used; it delivers an inadequate breakthrough dose, is painful and reduces the time of infusion.

Chapter 5

Mouth care

Julie Hewett

Pre-reading exercise 5.1
Time: 30 minutes

Test your knowledge of oral health.

1 What is xerostomia?
2 List five causes of poor oral health in palliative care patients.
3 A patient is complaining of a sore mouth. List three possible reasons for this.
4 Name three items of equipment you should have to perform an oral assessment.
5 Name three qualities of life that are affected by a sore, dirty, dry mouth.

(*See* answers on page 102.)

Introduction

The importance to quality of life of a healthy, comfortable mouth is highly relevant to the care of all patients. However, for the patient with cancer, oral health is integral to care.[1] Mouth care may appear minor in comparison to the patient's diagnosis and prognosis. Self-esteem and motivation can be raised by ensuring that the mouth is pain-free and clean.[2] Many patients undergoing palliative treatments suffer mouth problems.[3] In a hospice environment, a wide range of oral symptoms are encountered (*see* Box 5.1).

Box 5.1 Oral symptoms encountered in palliative care[4]

- Xerostomia (dry mouth) (64%).
- Erythema (cause unknown) (68%).
- Oral candidosis (44%).
- Disturbance of taste (4%).
- Soreness (48%).
- Denture problems (12%).
- Coated tongue (48%).
- Ulceration (32%).
- Angular cheilitis (20%).
- Difficulty speaking (4%).

A government initiative[5] provides a benchmarking on oral hygiene. Care should be:

- negotiated with the patient
- based on an assessment of individual and clinical needs
- provided when required
- continuously evaluated and reassessed.

Effects of poor oral health

Patients may be embarrassed by bad breath and difficulty speaking, becoming withdrawn and isolated. Patients with a sore mouth may have dry lips that crack when smiling, laughing or kissing. A sore, dry mouth affects taste and food enjoyment. These are critical social activities and can result in interference with personal relationships[1] and support networks. In the older, infirm person, poor oral hygiene can predispose chest infection.[6]

Definition and aim of good mouth care

The principal objectives of mouth care for the patient who is very ill are to:

- keep the lining of the mouth and lips clean and soft[7]
- keep the oral mucosa moist
- prevent infection[8]
- alleviate halitosis and tooth decay by removing plaque and debris[7]
- promote patient comfort and quality of life.

There are many possible reasons for the interruption of these vital processes (*see* Box 5.2). Neglect of oral hygiene results in the fermentation of plaque. If untreated, this may lead to infection and breakdown of the oral mucosal lining.[9]

Box 5.2   Causes of poor oral health in palliative care patients

- Malnutrition, dysphagia, dehydration and deficiency of iron, protein, and vitamins B and C.
- Cytotoxic chemotherapy.
- Radiotherapy and brachytherapy.
- Myelosuppressed or otherwise immunocompromised patients.
- Surgery to the mouth.
- Local tumours.
- Antibiotic therapy.
- Anxiety, depression and pain.
- Oxygen therapy.
- Nausea and vomiting.

Oral assessment

Oral assessment is an essential component of effective and appropriate oral healthcare.[4] Oral assessment should be performed during the first encounter with the patient. Daily assessment is recommended for inpatients.[4] Ideally, assessment should be performed by the same professional to avoid subjectivity.

Key tip 5.1

Before beginning oral assessment:

- wash your hands
- put on gloves
- remove any dental appliances.

Always have:

- working pen torch
- tongue depressor
- dental mirror
- suction – if there is a choking or aspiration risk.[10]

Examination and assessment of the patient's oral cavity must be made, and can be scored according to findings (*see* Box 5.3). Frequency of care is determined according to the final score.

A mouth-care treatment regime, conducted 3–4 hourly, or after meals and before bedtime, is recommended to reduce the potential risk of infection by microorganisms.[10–12] For the patient with stomatitis (inflammation of the mouth) or gingivitis (inflammation of the gums), anaemia may be problematic.[2] The frequency of mouth care should be 2-hourly to reduce oral complications and maintain patient comfort and cleanliness, with 1-hourly moisturising of the mouth if the patient is:

- severely ill
- unconscious
- mouth breathing
- receiving oxygen[1] – oxygen should always be humidified

or where oral infection is involved.[12]

Patient and family involvement

Over 90% of patients with cancer spend the last year of life at home with the family as carers and district nurses supporting those carers.[13] However, it cannot be assumed that the family are comfortable with the term carer, or attribute the term to themselves.[14] Involving the family can be positive. It can reduce their sense of isolation and powerlessness.[15]

It is not acceptable for the family to learn by 'trial and error.' Therefore, it is important to ensure that individualised information and teaching are provided and that understanding is frequently assessed.[16]

Box 5.3   Mouth-care assessment record

Reproduced with the kind permission of South Devon Health Care NHS Trust. Anning P, Lye P. *Adult Assessment Tool and Intervention Standards for Mouthcare*. Torquay: South Devon Healthcare NHS Trust, Torbay Hospital; July 2005.

	Initial assessment					Review assessments				
Date of oral assessment										
Voice 1 = Normal 2 = Deeper/raspy 3 = Difficult/painful speech										
Ability to swallow 1 = Normal swallow 2 = Some pain on swallow 3 = Unable to swallow										
Lips 1 = Smooth/pink/moist 2 = Dry/cracked 3 = Ulcerated or bleeding										
Tongue 1 = Pink/moist/papillae present 2 = Coated or less of papillae 3 = Blistered or cracked										
Saliva 1 = Watery 2 = Thick or ropey 3 = Absent										
Mucous/membranes 1 = Pink/moist 2 = Red/inflamed/coated 3 = Very red/blistered or ulcerated										
Gingiva 1 = Pink/moist 2 = Oedematous/red 3 = Red shiny/ulcerated or bleeding										
Teeth/dentures 1 = Clean/no debris 2 = Dull, localised plaque 3 = Very dull, generalised plaque/debris										
Candida 0 – No 2 – Yes – refer to doctor										
Oral assessment score										
Review date										
Nurse's initials										
Other problems noted										

This assessment is intended as a guide to improve mouth care

SCORE	ACTION
1–8 Basic care	• Able to use own toothpaste and toothbrush themselves and no problem identified.
9–10 Intermediate care	• Continued encouragement of basic care. • Twice daily mouthwash of Thymol or Corsodyl® if prescribed. • If mild pain or discomfort is experienced, Difflam mouthwash can be prescribed four times a day in conjunction with the above. • Where patients with learning disabilities are being managed, dental referral may be appropriate. • If persistent pain continues, ensure adequate analgesia is prescribed, e.g. paracetamol. • Advise the removal of dentures if pain/discomfort or bleeding is present. • Re-assess nutritional score and consider referral to a dietician. • Maintain appropriate fluid intake • Re-assessment should be carried out once a day and recorded on the assessment record sheet.
11 or more Advanced care	• Continue with intermediate care. • Consider referral to ENT or dental services, if appropriate. • Increase pain management interventions using pain assessment tool and discuss with medical staff. • Re-assessment should be carried out at least once a day or more frequently if required and recorded on the assessment record sheet. *NB: If patient is unconscious assess their mouth-care requirements using the tool and undertake nursing intervention as appropriate.*

A gentle approach

Mouth treatment is a personal concern, especially when handled by another person. Consent is essential, using a gentle, caring and respectful approach.

Tools for oral care

Toothbrush

The toothbrush provides the most effective means of cleaning teeth, removing plaque and debris.[12,16] Use a small, soft, round-ended toothbrush. Brush all tooth surfaces. Thick tongue coating can be gently brushed, if the tongue is not too sore. Clean dentures the same way.[16]

> **Key tip 5.2**
> - Do not store toothbrushes in a toilet bag.
> - Allow toothbrush to air dry.
> - Replace every 6–12 weeks.[11]

Foam sticks

Use *a foam stick* if the patient's condition prevents the use of a toothbrush, e.g. if spontaneous bleeding or pain is present. Foam sticks will not efficiently remove plaque,[17] but are effective in removing thick mucus and food debris. If they must be used, they are more effective in removing plaque if soaked in chlorhexidine.[18]

Toothpaste

Toothpaste contains fluoride which prevents cavity formation.[19] It is inexpensive, refreshing and effective in removing plaque, as long as the brushing technique is thorough. Use a pea-sized amount of toothpaste, and press into the brush surface to avoid inhalation.[1] Personal preferences vary but for sensitive teeth, a paste containing strontium chloride (e.g. Sensodyne®) can prevent painful stimuli from reaching exposed nerves.[19] Thorough rinsing with warm water is important as any toothpaste left in the mouth can have a drying effect. Biotene® oral toothpaste is formulated to relieve a dry mouth.

Dental floss

Floss daily. Flossing between the teeth helps prevent plaque and tartar. However, exercise care when using floss to keep gum trauma to a minimum.[16]

Cleansing agents

Warm saline mouthwashes

Saline mouthwashes can be made using 5 ml (1 teaspoonful) of salt to 500 ml (1 pint) of water.[19] Saline promotes healing and the formation of granulation tissue and does not irritate or taste unpleasant. It should be used four times a day.[16] A soothing and pain-free agent is likely to be used regularly.[13] Saline is useful in the care of mucositis, for irrigating a furred sore tongue, and for use after brushing the teeth as an effective mouth rinse.

Chlorhexidine 0.2% (Corsodyl®)

Antiseptic solutions containing chlorhexidine effectively reduce bacteria in 80% of patients.[1] In addition, it can prevent plaque formation on teeth[8,20] but causes staining. A dentist can remove this. If stinging or burning is caused, dilute it 50:50 with water.[2] Rinse 10 ml around the mouth for 1 minute twice daily after meals and tooth brushing.[2,20] Take nothing orally for 1 hour following the rinse. Chlorhexidine is available in gel form that can be applied directly to the teeth and gums. This is useful where there is any risk of aspiration with mouth rinsing.

Sodium bicarbonate

An inexpensive, widely available, alkaline cleansing agent that may be effective in dissolving tenacious mucus or a 'sloughy' mouth.[4,9] The recommended dilution is one 5 ml teaspoonful in 500 ml (1 pint) of water. It should be used four times a day.[2] However, it must be diluted correctly to avoid superficial burns.[21] Sodium bicarbonate helps reduce mouth odour but it tastes unpleasant[2] and has a negative effect on the oral mucosa, allowing bacteria to multiply.[22] Despite its wide use in oncology settings, there is no firm evidence to support its use in palliative care.

Vitamin C

Effervescent ascorbic acid (vitamin C) is widely used to loosen heavy mucus coating. The high sugar and citric acid contents of some tablets may have a detrimental effect on tooth enamel. In addition, repeated use can lower the pH of the mouth, promoting fungal growth. There is no conclusive evidence for its use.

Denture care

Denture care is an important aspect in care of the mouth. Dentures can be associated with many oral problems.[23] Denture stomatitis is an inflammatory condition of the mucosa, which is manifested as erythema of the tissues supporting the denture; this can cause pain and discomfort. *Candida albicans* is associated with most cases of denture stomatitis.[23] For denture stomatitis, cleanse and soak dentures in chlorhexidine mouthwash solution for 15 minutes twice daily.[20]

Denture dos and don'ts!

Dos

- Take dentures out at night.
- Store dentures in fresh cold Milton™ solution (*hot Milton™ solution may cause denture bleaching*). Change Milton daily.
- Remove dentures, brush and rinse after meals.
- Treat dentures with antifungal agents if the mouth is infected with *Candida* species.
- Check the dentures fit the gums and are not rubbing or causing mucosal trauma. Replace or alter as required.

Don'ts

- Wear dentures if the mouth is sore or infected.
- Soak metal dentures or those with a metal frame in Milton™ solution (corrosion risk). Instead, use chlorhexidine 0.2% (Corsodyl©).

- Use self-applied commercial soft linings and denture fixatives:
  - they may mask problems which need professional dental attention
  - they act as a medium for the rapid proliferation of micro-organisms, particularly yeasts.

Common oral complaints

The following require vigilant care. Adopt a team approach. Dentists and dental specialists have much to offer in ensuring proper dental care for palliative care patients.[24]

Adequate explanation to patient and family about the cause of the complaint may relieve anxiety.[13]

Xerostomia (a feeling of dryness in the mouth)

Xerostomia is a common oral symptom in advanced cancer.[4]

Causes

- *Radiotherapy to the head and neck.*
- *Dehydration.*
- *Depression.*
- *Anxiety.*
- *Oral infection.*
- *Commonly used drugs* (*see* Box 5.4). Check medication. Can the drugs be altered?

Box 5.4   Drugs causing xerostomia

- Anticholinergics, e.g. hyoscine, atropine.
- Antiemetics, e.g. cyclizine, stemetil.
- Antibiotics – some.
- Anticonvulsants, e.g. phenytoin.
- Antidepressants, e.g. amitriptyline.
- Antihistamines.
- Antihypertensives, e.g. clonidine, methyldopa, lisinopril.
- Antineoplastics.
- Antimuscarinics for parkinsonism.
- Antipsychotics, e.g. chlorpromazine.
- Bronchodilators.
- Diuretics.
- Narcotic analgesics.
- Steroids.

Treatment

Avoid sugary foods. A dry mouth loses the normal protective functions of saliva (*see* Box 5.5) and consequently the patient's teeth may decay and s/he may develop oral thrush.[14]

Box 5.5   Some wonders of saliva!

- It moistens and lubricates food, and aids bolus formation.
- It cleanses the mouth and teeth of cellular debris.
- Lysozymes present in saliva help to control and destroy bacteria.
- Saliva produces a neutral pH, which prevents cavity formation in teeth.
- It acts as a solvent in which food molecules can be dissolved and thus tasted.

The following may be useful measures:

- *Pilocarpine (a muscarinic antagonist)* – 5 mg three times a day with or immediately after food.[13,20,25] Administration may be burdened by potential side effects. Do *not* use with a diagnosis of:
  - asthma
  - COPD
  - bradycardia
  - renal or hepatic impairment
  - bowel obstruction
  - angle-closure glaucoma.[20]
- *Artificial saliva* – as required, e.g. Luborant®, Saliva Orthana®, Salivace®, Saliveze®, or Glandosane® sprays, Salivix® pastilles, SST tablets.[20]
- *Salivary peroxidase-based* – gel, toothpaste and mouthwash, e.g. Biotene Oralbalance®, BioXtra®.
- *Jugs of iced water, chips.*[26]
- *Sucking* – raw jelly, sugar-free sweets or ice lollies.
- *Encourage* – increase in unsweetened fluids.[9,11]
- *Pineapple* – suck provided the mouth is not sore. This is a natural saliva stimulant.[27] Contains the enzyme *ananase* which cleans the mouth.[9,25]
- *Sugar-free gum* – a salivary stimulant, e.g. Endekay™. Sixty per cent of patients prefer chewing gum to the use of artificial saliva.[28] Chew one or two pieces gently, using both sides of the mouth, for 10 minutes.[29]
- *Coat lip* – with white or yellow soft paraffin,[15] Biotene® oral gel or a light moisturising cream. Clean first with normal saline.
- *Alter diet* – include foods with a high moisture content (consult a dietician).
- *Acupuncture* – potentially palliates xerostomia.[30] Acupuncture may improve xerostomia with an increase in the salivary flow rate.[31] Eighty-one per cent of head and neck cancer patients, with post-radiotherapy xerostomia, report an improvement in their perceived levels of oral dryness.[32]

Oral thrush

Candidiasis is the most common fungal infection.[33] It manifests as a:

- white-yellowish plaque that can easily be removed, leaving a bleeding, painful surface[33]
- red, smooth mucosa, smooth tongue and angular cheilitis.

Infection may be due to the immunocompromised state of patients with advanced cancer, often in conjunction with xerostomia.[34]

Treatment

Treatment includes:

- *Fluconazole* – 50–100mg daily for 7–14 days:[12]
  - prolonged or repeated exposure may be associated with the emergence of fluconazole-resistant strains[34]
  - a larger single dose is especially useful if the patient has a short time to live.
- *Nystatin suspension* – 100 000 U/ml four times daily after food,[20] held in the mouth for 2–3 minutes before swallowing:[35]
  - do not rinse or take food/drink for 1 hour after treatment
  - soak dentures in nystatin overnight to reduce/remove risk of re-infection from the plastic, which may harbour the candida[36]
  - chlorhexidine mouth rinses may also reduce infection
  - remove dentures before treatment and 30 minutes after chlorhexidine is used[12]
  - replace toothbrushes after fungal infection.[13]
- *Miconazole gel* – via a foam stick directly to the oral cavity four times a day:[37]
  - helpful for the unconscious patient
  - if angular cheilitis is present, use miconazole gel topically four times daily to the corners of the mouth[12]
  - can be used in conjunction with an antibacterial cream, such as Bactroban®, because co-infection by *Candida albicans* and *Staphylococcus aureus* is common[12]
  - apply miconazole oral gel to denture before insertion (*short periods only*).[20]

Painful mouth

Oral pain causes suffering disproportionate to the size of the area affected due to the proliferation of sensory nerve endings in the mouth. Systemic analgesia may be required to treat oral pain, including the use of opioids.[35] In palliative care:

- Morphine may be given continually, subcutaneously, via a syringe driver:[2]
  - topical morphine can be useful (0.3–0.5%) in intracite gel for mucositis.[25]
- Mouth pain, commonly due to mouth ulcers, can be helped by benzydamine mouthwash (Difflam® – 0.15%), a locally acting analgesic with anti-inflammatory properties:
  - used as an oral rinse every 3 hours (dilute with water 50:50 if stings)
  - used for up to 7 days[13]
  - can be given in a spray form[17]

- use Difflam[®] for the treatment of oral mucositis caused by radiotherapy and chemotherapy.[38]
- Mouth ulcers can be treated with Orabase paste[®].[3,13] This forms a protective coat over mucosal surfaces and relieves painful ulcers on the tongue, gums and mucous membranes:
  - recommended dosage – apply twice daily for 1 week[39]
  - soluble aspirin rinses and oxetacaine or mucaine – useful during early stages of stomatitis
  - sucralfate, an anti-ulcer drug – eases painful, ulcerated mouth by binding to ulcerated tissue, creating a protective coating[16,17]
  - choline salicylate gel (Bonjela gel[®]) – effective for mouth ulcers, but can cause stinging and pain on application[35]
  - Gelclair[®] – an oral protective rinse.[40]
- If chronic ulceration persists, or if the patient has a local tumour, an anaerobic antibiotic, e.g. metronidazole syrup (200 mg every 8 hours for 3–7 days[20]) can be useful.[33]

Conclusion

Oral discomfort and pain is distressing and often inadequately dealt with, in a ritualised manner, by the professional.[3,22,27,37,39] Managing oral pain enables the maintenance of oral care, nutritional status and, ultimately, the prognosis of the patient.[41]

The state of the mouth is indicative of the level of nursing care received.[9] For long-term palliative patients, the ability to:

- converse freely
- smile
- laugh
- taste and enjoy food

is essential. This is the essence of maintaining a good quality of life. Patients with cancer may experience a variety of feelings, e.g. anxiety, fear, loss of self-esteem and control. However, if the individual is involved in his or her mouth care, self-worth and confidence will increase.[9]

An oral assessment tool is helpful in monitoring the individual's holistic needs.[3] However, tools and agents for care must be employed carefully. The mouth should *never* be neglected. It is of equal importance to other areas that perhaps have a higher profile in palliative care. In addition, dentists and dental specialists have a pivotal role in ensuring proper oral management for palliative care patients, maintaining comfort and eliminating sites of infection or potential infection.[24]

Acknowledgement

I would like to acknowledge the work produced by my good friend and early mentor Elizabeth (Libby) Potter in the mouth-care chapter for the first edition. I have been able to utilise some of the hard work she put in at that time, adding to it my own findings from some of the most recent research and publications available.

References

1 Rawlins C, Trueman I. Effective mouth care for seriously ill patients. *Professional Nurse*. 2001; **16**(4): 1025–1028.

2 Denton E. Palliative care: mouth care an indicator of the level of nursing care a patient receives? *Journal Community Nursing*. 1999; **13**(11): www.jcn.co.uk.

3 Wood A. Mouth care and ritualistic practice. *Can Nurs Practice*. 2004; **3**(4): 34–39.

4 Milligan S, McGill M, Sweeney M *et al*. Oral care for people with advanced cancer: an evidence based protocol. *Int J Pall Nurs*. 2001; **7**(9): 418–426.

5 Department of Health. *The Essence of Care: benchmarks for personal and oral hygiene*. NHS Modernisation Agency. London: Department of Health Publishing; 2001.

6 Loesch W, Schork A, Terpenning M *et al*. Assessing the relationship between dental disease and coronary heart disease in elderly US veterans. *J Am Dent Assoc*. 1988; **129**(3): 310–311.

7 Doyle D, Hanks G, MacDonald N. *Oxford Textbook of Palliative Medicine*. Oxford: Oxford University Press; 1996.

8 Evans G. A rationale for oral care. *Nursing Standard*. 2001; **15**(43): 33–36.

9 Heals D. A key to wellbeing: oral hygiene in patients with advanced cancer. *Professional Nurse*. 1993; **8**(6) 391–398.

10 Curzio J, McCowan M. Getting research into practice: developing oral hygiene standards. *BJN*. 2000; **9**(7): 434–438.

11 Jones C. The importance of oral hygiene in nutritional support. *BJN*. 1998; **7**(2): 74–83.

12 Lanarkshire Palliative Care Guidelines Committee. *Palliative Care Guidelines*. St Andrew's Lanarkshire: St Andrew's Hospice; 2005: www.lcis.org.uk.

13 Feber T. *Head and Neck Oncology Nursing*. London: Whurr Publishers Ltd; 2000.

14 Payne S, Seymour J, Ingleton C. *Palliative Care Nursing: principles and evidence for practice*. Berkshire: Open University Press; 2004.

15 Eldridge AD. Mouthcare technique promotes patient comfort. *Oncol Nurse Forum*. 1993; **20**: 700.

16 Hanson C. Mouth care – how important is it? *J Comm Nursing*. 2004; **18**(8): 4–8.

17 Pearson L, Hutton J. A controlled trial to compare the ability of foam swabs and toothbrushes to remove dental plaque. *Journal of Advanced Nursing*. 2002; **39**(5): 480–489.

18 Barker G, Epstein J, Williams K *et al*. Current practice and knowledge of oral care for cancer patients: a survey of supportive healthcare providers. *Support Care Cancer*. 2005; **13**(32): 32–41.

19 Madeya M. Oral complications from cancer therapy. Part 2. Nursing implications for assessment and treatment. *Oncol Nurses Forum*. 1996; **23**: 808–818.

20 British Medical Association and Royal Pharmaceutical Society of Great Britain. *British National Formulary*. London: British Medical Association and Royal Pharmaceutical Society of Great Britain; 2004.

21 Howarth H. Mouthcare procedures for the very ill. *Nursing Times*. 1997; **83**: 25–27.

22 Miller M, Kearney N. Oral care for patients with cancer: a review of the literature. *Cancer Nursing*. 2001; **24**(4): 241–254.

23 Finegan W. *HELP (Helpful Essential Links to Palliative Care)*, 3rd edition. Dundee: Macmillan Cancer Relief/Centre for Macmillan Education, University of Dundee; 1999.

24 Chiodo G, Tolle S, Madden T. The dentist's role in end-of-life care. *General Dentistry*. 1998; **46**(6): 560–565.

25 Twycross R. *Introducing Palliative Care*, 4th edition. Oxford: Radcliffe Medical Press; 2003.

26 Clarkson J, Worthington H, Eden O. Interventions for preventing oral mucositis for patients with cancer receiving treatment. Cochrane Review. *The Cochrane Library issue 3*. York: University of York; 2003.

27 Freer S. Use of an oral assessment tool to improve practice. *Professional Nurse*. 2000; **15**(10): 635–637.

28 Bots C, Brand H, Veerman E *et al*. The management of xerostomia in patients on haemodialysis: a comparison of artificial saliva and chewing gum. *Palliative Medicine*. 2005; **19**(3): 202–207.

29 Davies A. A comparison of artificial saliva and chewing gum in the management of xerostomia in patients with advanced cancer. *Palliative Medicine*. 2000; **14**: 197–203.

30   Johnstone P, Niemtzow R, Riffenburgh R. Acupuncture for xerostomia. *Cancer*. 2002; **94**: 1151–1156 .

31   Neimtzow R, May B, Peng Y *et al*. *Acupuncture Technique for Pilocarpine Resistant Xerostomia Following Radiotherapy for Head and Neck Malignancies*. 2002; www.n5ev.com/art_ pilocarpine.htm

32   Hewett J, Singam S. *Acupuncture for Patients with Xerostomia Following Radiotherapy to the Head and Neck*. Unpublished pilot study. South Devon Healthcare Trust. Torquay: Torbay Hospital; 2004.

33   Veniafridda V, Ripamonti C, Sbanatto A *et al*. Mouthcare. In: Doyle D, Flanks G, MacDonald N, editors. *Oxford Textbook of Palliative Medicine*. Oxford: Oxford Medical Publications; 1993.

34   Bagg J, Sweeny M, Lewis M *et al*. High prevalence of non-albicans yeasts and detection of anti-fungal resistance in the oral flora of patients with advanced cancer. *Palliative Medicine*. 2003; **17**(6): 477–481.

35   Finlay I. Oral fungal infections. *Eur J Palliative Care Suppl.* 1995; **2**: 4–7.

36   Groenwald S, Hansen Frogge M, Goodman M *et al*. *Cancer Nursing, principles and practice*, 4th edition. London: Jones and Bartlett; 1997.

37   Fife Area Drug and Therapeutics Committee. *Fife Palliative Care Guidelines*; 2004: www. scan.scot.nhs.uk.

38   Epstein J. Oropharyngeal mucositis in cancer therapy. Review of pathogenesis, diagnosis and management. *Oncology (Huntington)*. 2003; **17**(12): 1767–1779.

39   Charlton R, editor. *Primary Palliative Care – dying, death and bereavement in the community*. Oxford: Radcliffe Medical Press; 2002.

40   Innocenti M, Moscatelli G, Copez S. Efficacy of gelclair in reducing pain in palliative care patients with oral lesions: preliminary findings from an open pilot. *J Pain Sym Man*. 2002; **24**(5): 456–457.

41   Cooley C. Oral health: basic or essential? *Cancer Nursing Practice*. 2002; 1(3): 33–39

To learn more

- Fife Area Drug and Therapeutics Committee. *Fife Oral Care Guidelines for Patients with Cancer and Palliative Care*; 2004: www.scan.scot.nhs.uk.
- Huda Abu-Saad. *Evidence Based Palliative Care: across the life span*. London: Blackwell Science; 2001.
- O'Connor M, Aranda S, editors. *Palliative Care Nursing: a guide to practice*, 2nd edition. Oxford: Radcliffe Medical Press; 2003.
- Regnard CFB, Tempest S. *A Guide to Symptom Relief in Advanced Disease*, 4th edition. Manchester: Hochland and Hochland; 1998.
- Richardson A. *Manual of Core Care Plans for Cancer Nursing*, 1st edition. London: The Royal Marsden Hospital, Scutari Press and Royal College of Nursing; 1992.
- Lanarkshire Palliative Care Guidelines Committee. *Palliative Care Guidelines*. Lanarkshire: St Andrew's Hospice; 2005: www.lcis.org.uk.
- Sweeny M, Bagg J. *Making Sense of the Mouth: partnership in oral care*. Sponsored by Pfizer Ltd. Birmingham: Partnership in Oral Care; 1997.
- Twycross R, Wilcock A. *Symptom Management in Advanced Cancer*, 3rd edition. Oxford: Radcliffe Medical Press; 2001.

Complementary chapters

See also Stepping into Palliative Care 1: relationships and responses

- Chapter 11: The value of teamwork

See also Stepping into Palliative Care 2: care and practice

- Chapter 1: Assessment in palliative care
- Chapter 2: Introduction to pain management
- Chapter 12: Hearing the pain of the carer

Answers to Pre-reading exercise 5.1

1 Dry mouth.
2 Chemotherapy, radiotherapy, anxiety, depression and malnutrition.
3 Oral thrush, mouth ulcers and dry mouth.
4 Pen torch, tongue depressor, gloves and, if possible, a dental mirror.
5 Talking, taste, kissing, eating.

Chapter 6

Lymphoedema

Annie Hogg

Pre-reading exercise 6.1
Time: 30 minutes

Reflect on a patient you have cared for where tissue swelling was a significant problem.

                  THINK! – physical – psychological – emotional – spiritual.

Consider:

- What impact did the tissue swelling have on the patient?
- How effectively was the swelling assessed?
- What interventions (if any) were introduced?
- Were they effective?

After reading this chapter:

- Consider any changes you might make in the future.
- Identify the rationale for these changes.

Introduction

Oedema of the limbs, trunk and genitalia is a common and often significant symptom of advanced cancer. Despite this, lymphoedema, and its management, is poorly understood and a neglected aspect of palliative care.

This chapter aims to promote understanding and enhance skills, reducing the significant effects of oedema in advanced disease.

What is oedema?

Oedema is an excessive accumulation of fluid in the interstitial compartment of the tissues resulting from an imbalance between capillary filtration and lymph drainage.

Causes

In advanced cancer, several concurrent factors may contribute to the formation of oedema. For example, in advanced pelvic malignant disease, lymph node infiltration and inferior vena cava compression may cause leg swelling, possibly compounded by:

- hypoproteinaemia
- anaemia
- immobility.[1]

General causes

- End stage renal failure.
- Drugs which cause vasodilation.
- Drugs which cause salt and water retention.
- Malignant ascites.
- Cardiac failure (+/– anaemia).
- Hypoproteinaemia.

Local causes

- Venous obstruction.
- Lymphatic obstruction/damage – due to radiotherapy, surgery, tumour in lymph nodes.
- Lymphovenousoedema – due to immobility and dependence.

Assessment

The goal of oedema management comprises:

- reduction
- control
- palliation.

This varies according to where the patient is along the cancer journey. Effective assessment of oedema in palliative care must establish what impact the oedema has on the quality of life, and what interventions can be modified to meet the individual needs. If the patient is in good health, active intervention may be acceptable and appropriate. However, if the patient is very poorly, active intervention may not be appropriate.

Assessment includes:

- medical history
- clinical signs and symptoms
- psychological and psychosocial assessment.

Medical history

Past and current medical history will help establish the cause of the oedema. Knowledge of the

- site of disease
- treatment
- current disease status
- medications

may indicate local or general causes of oedema and contributory factors. A history of swelling presentation and any changes may indicate how reversible the swelling is.

Clinical signs and symptoms

This requires:

- a physical examination of the affected and surrounding area
- careful questioning regarding physical effects
- condition and integrity of the skin
- presence of any infective or inflammatory process
- extent of the swelling
- distortion of shape.

The presence of:

- pain – a significant feature of oedema affecting up to 50% of patients
- discomfort
- tightness
- heaviness
- impairment of function and/or mobility – as a result of the swelling.

Psychological and psychosocial assessment

Psychological and psychosocial assessment explores the impact and influence the swelling has on the *whole* person:

- what does it mean
- altered body image
- disease reminder
- fear of recurrence
- visible symptom of cancer – reaction of family and friends
- impact of limitation of function and mobility on vocational, domestic, social and sexual life
- problems with clothing and footwear.

Management

The four main components of care are:

- skin care
- exercise and movement

- massage
- external support/compression.

The aim to reduce, control or palliate the symptoms will be determined by the patient's general health and care needs and their priorities.

Reduction and control

Unless there are correctable causes for the swelling, there is no curative treatment for oedema. However, in certain circumstances, it is possible to enhance drainage of fluid, thereby significantly reducing and controlling the swelling. If the patient is too frail to tolerate reduction, it may be possible to prevent the oedema increasing.

Skin care

Aimed at:

- improving the condition of dermis and epidermis so they are hydrated, intact, and supple[3]
- reducing the risk of infection.

Action:

- daily thorough skin hygiene
- daily skin moisturising – using bland emollients, e.g. aqueous cream
- avoiding skin damage
- prompt treatment of injuries
- advice on wearing well-fitting, comfortable shoes and clothes.

Exercise and movement

Aimed at:

- encouraging lymph flow
- maintaining muscle tone
- improving joint mobility and function.[4]

Action:

- normal use of the limb is encouraged, if tolerated
- specific exercise tailored to the patient's ability and general condition
- avoid static activities if possible – they may increase swelling
- passive movements.

Massage

Aimed at:

- stimulating lymph drainage away from the congested area.

Action:

- *manual lymph drainage* – specialised massage performed by a trained therapist

- *self-massage* – an adaptation of the above which can be administered by the patient or carer.

External support/compression

Aimed at:

- promoting lymph drainage
- relieving tension and tightness
- reducing and/or controlling swelling.

Action:

- *multilayer compression bandaging*
- *elastic compression garments.*

Palliative management

Correct the correctable

- Anaemia.
- Fluid-retaining drugs.
- Malignant ascites.
- Anti-cancer treatment.

Oedema in advanced disease can result in a variety of problems. It is unlikely that the degree of swelling will be reduced.

Action:

- relieve discomfort
- enhance quality of life
- prevent deterioration.

Symptoms associated with oedema

- Skin problems.
- Truncal swelling.
- Pain.
- Impaired function and mobility.

Skin problems

- Infection – acute inflammatory incident/fungal.
- Dry/thin/fragile skin.
- Ulceration.
- Lymphorrhoea.

Action:

- *The basic components of skin care (as above) remain an important element in maintaining skin integrity.*

- *Inflammation/infection* – antibiotics/topical antifungal preparations.
- *Dry/fragile skin* – avoid use of elastic compression garments as they may cause further damage.
- *Ulceration/lesions* – appropriate non-adherent dressings secured by a light bandage.
- *Lymphorrhoea* – leakage of lymph fluid can be profuse and often distressing and difficult to manage, particularly in the home setting. Gentle pressure applied by means of palliative bandaging or Tubigrip® appears to be the most widely used method of treatment where comfort is pivotal. Use of padding or incontinence sheets, and frequent dressing changes are necessary to maintain comfort and dignity.

Truncal swelling

Swelling may extend beyond the roof of a limb involving the trunk and genitalia. This can be extremely distressing and incapacitating. Compression may enhance lymph drainage and reduce swelling. Some manufacturers make ready- or custom-made low compression garments but they are costly, and may take time to customise. Inventive measures may be more practical and readily available, such as the following.

Action:

- *Cycling shorts.*
- *Double layer support underwear.*
- *Insertion of sanitary towels inside underpants.*
- *Maternity garments.*
- *Support tights.*

Compression of the adjacent limb may increase truncal and genital swelling. Massage to improve lymph flow from the genitalia and lower trunk may reduce this.

Pain

- Myofascial.
- Infection/inflammation.
- Arthropathies/bursitis.
- Neuropathic.

Pain is a common and complex problem. The burden of a heavy, swollen limb, possibly exacerbated by infection, inflammation, and infiltration or pressure on nerves, can result in distressing pain sensations. Function and mobility are likely to be further impeded by the presence of pain.

A range of pharmacological and non-pharmacological interventions may be required. The interdisciplinary approach, encompassing nurse, physiotherapist, occupational therapist and palliative care team, will provide the opportunity for optimum benefit to the patient. Good and effective communication between professionals is vital in optimising care for the patient and family. Decisions on care need to be interdisciplinary, with the lead and final decision coming from the patient.

Action:

- *Pharmacological*:
  - *analgesia*:
    - *non-opioids*
    - *opioids*
    - *anti-inflammatories*
  - *adjuvant analgesia*:
    - *antidepressants*
    - *anticonvulsants*
    - *corticosteroids*
  - *muscle relaxants*
  - *antibiotics.*

Diuretics can be advantageous if there is a cardiac or venous component. Furosemide (frusemide) can be prescribed for a 1-week trial and reviewed. Consider a 1-week trial of dexamethasone 4–8 mg. By reducing peri-tumour oedema, lymphatic obstruction may be reduced. [5]

- *Non-pharmacological*:
  - *explore patient's fears and worries* – assessment and questioning is pivotal to good management; the emotional impact of altered body image may not be immediately obvious
  - *explanation to reduce psychological impact of pain* – careful **listening** and truly **hearing** what the pain means to that person can enable the professional to explain the process, at a level that meets individual needs
  - *TENS* – may help to reduce pain
  - *positioning* – support with pillows and/or specially made foam: splints/supports, elevation of legs when sat, broad arm sling when ambulant
  - *containment support bandaging* – can be taught to carers/relatives, shaped Tubigrip®, low compression hosiery
  - *passive movements to reduce stiffness and discomfort.*

Impaired function and mobility

Action:

- *Aids for walking and dressing.*
- *Special cutlery for swollen/weak hands and arms.*
- *Pain management.*
- *Passive movements.*
- *Consider occupational therapy assessment.*

The skills of occupational therapists and physiotherapists are invaluable.

Key tip 6.1

An occupational therapist utilised students from a local engineering college to custom build a raised wheeled trolley to support a grossly swollen arm, enabling the patient to retain some mobility at home.

Conclusion

Oedema can affect the individual in many ways. Significant reduction and control can be achieved when active treatment is appropriate. It is important to remember the needs of the patient and family, to establish the level of understanding.

The palliative care of oedema is complex. The resultant physical disabilities and symptomology require innovative and imaginative solutions to enhance patients' quality of life.

All members of the interdisciplinary team make an important contribution. Care is often labour intensive and predominantly carried out at home by the carer. This degree of physical care can be enriching for some carers enabling maintenance of physical contact and reduce the feeling of helplessness. However, the burden of care can be enormous, and individuals' resources limited in the presence of the many difficulties.

Professionals must collaborate with the patient and family by:

- *being sensitive to needs*
- *providing empathetic intervention and support*
- *maintaining a therapeutic and helping relationship.*

Self-assessment exercise 6.1
Time: 15 minutes

1 What cancer treatments may lead to the development of oedema?
2 What are the three possible goals of oedema management?
3 What constitutes the assessment process?
4 Name three main goals of palliative management of oedema.

(*See* answers on page 111.)

References

1 Keeley V. Oedema in advanced cancer. In: Twycross R, Jenns K, Todd J, editors. *Lymphoedema.* Oxford: Radcliffe Medical Press; 2000.
2 Carroll D, Rose K. Treatment leads to significant improvement: effect of conservative treatment on pain in lymphoedema. *Professional Nurse.* 1992; **8**(1): 32–36.
3 Williams AC. Update: lymphoedema. *Professional Nurse.* 1997; **12**(9): 645–648.
4 Miller LT. Exercise in the management of breast cancer related lymphoedema. *Innovations in Breast Cancer Care.* 1998; **3**(4): 101–106.
5 Twycross R, Wilcock A. *Symptom Management in Advanced Cancer,* 3rd edition. Oxford: Radcliffe Medical Press; 2001.

To learn more

- British Lymphology Society. *Chronic Oedema Population and Needs.* Sevenoaks, Kent: British Lymphology Society; 2001.
- Twycross R, Jenns K, Todd J, editors. *Lymphoedema.* Oxford: Radcliffe Medical Press; 2000.
- Twycross R, Wilcock A. *Symptom Management in Advanced Cancer,* 3rd edition. Oxford: Radcliffe Medical Press; 2001.

Complementary chapters

See also Stepping into Palliative Care 1: relationships and responses

- Chapter 3: The cancer journey
- Chapter 4: The experience of illness
- Chapter 5: The psychological impact of serious illness
- Chapter 6: Hope and coping strategies
- Chapter 7: The therapeutic relationship
- Chapter 11: The value of teamwork
- Chapter 15: Transcultural and ethnic issues at the end of life
- Chapter 16: Sexuality and palliative care

See also Stepping into Palliative Care 2: care and practice

- Chapter 1: Assessment in pallaitve care
- Chapter 2: Introduction to pain management
- Chapter 3: Symptom management: a framework
- Chapter 12: Hearing the pain of the carer
- Chapter 13: Spirituality and palliative care

Answers to Self-assessment exercise 6.1

1 Surgery, radiotherapy.
2 Reduction, control, palliation.
3 Medical history – clinical signs and symptoms – psychological and psycho-social assessment.
4 Relieve discomfort, enhance quality of life, prevent deterioration.

Chapter 7

Wound care

Mark Collier

Pre-reading exercise 7.1
Time: 30 minutes

- Reflect on a patient whom you recently cared for who had a malignant fungating lesion.
- Write brief notes relating to the specific wound management inter-ventions that you either undertook or observed another professional undertake on the patient's behalf.
- Ask a colleague to do the same.
- Discuss and compare your notes.

Introduction

This chapter introduces several aspects of wound care that are important to understand if we are to effectively undertake an overall, specific and holistic assessment and the management of patients with malignant (fungating) lesions.

Key tip 7.1

Fungating malignant wounds are visible markers of an underlying disease.[1]

The term fungating wounds refer to the infiltration into, and proliferation of, malignant cells through the epidermis of the skin. The origin may be a local tumour, or a distant primary lesion due to metastatic activity.[2] These tumours may grow rapidly and often take on a cauliflower-like appearance. However, they may also ulcerate and form shallow craters that can be complicated by the presence of an associated sinus or fistula.[3] Because of the amount of wound exudate that is normally associated with the latter group, these are commonly described as *malodorous* wounds.

A malodorous wound may be defined as *any wound assessed as being offensive (smelly) by either the patient and/or the professional*. Nevertheless, it is important to remember that a variety of wound aetiologies (e.g. pressure ulcers, leg ulcers, traumatic wounds) can be malodorous without being malignant, whereas in the majority of cases fungating wounds will have an associated odour assessed at some point during their treatment.[4]

Key tip 7.2

Knowledge of the epidemiology and pathophysiology of fungating lesions will assist the professionals' communication with the patient and family, and anticipate the likely issue that may be encountered if the disease process is not addressed adequately.

Epidemiology

UK epidemiological studies are rare, with most reported data being based on estimations.[5] However, one retrospective survey, utilising information collected mainly from radiotherapy and oncology units, discussed the most reliable data.[6] Respondents were asked to:

- record how many fungating wounds they had seen over the previous 4 weeks
- indicate whether the resultant figure was typical of an average month
- estimate how many cases of this particular wound type they had encountered during the previous year.

Of the 114 responses, a monthly total of 295 fungating wounds was reported, with an annual total of 2417. In addition, the location of fungating wounds was as follows:

- breast 62%
- head and face 24%
- groin and genitals 3%
- back 3%
- others 8%.

Pathophysiology

Tumour infiltration of the skin involves the spread of malignant cells along pathways that offer minimal resistance including:

- tissue planes
- blood and lymph capillaries
- perineural spaces.[7]

Abnormalities in the vascularisation of the lesion and surrounding tissues are often associated with tumour formation, although the mechanisms involved in the control of this process are not yet fully understood. However, hypoxic regions within the margins of the tumour will occur as a result of fluctuations in the blood supply and cell perfusion. Deficiencies may arise in the lymphatic system, affecting interstitial tissue drainage when interstitial fluid pressures exceed extravascular pressures and lead to the collapse of vessel walls. Therefore, the haemostasis of blood, lymph, interstitial and cellular environments may be severely disturbed.[3] For example, rapid proliferation of tumour cells may occur in the acidic pH conditions of extracellular fluid, which in turn will affect the tension within the blood cells.[8]

Tissue hypoxia in a fungating wound can be a significant problem, as anaerobic organisms flourish in accessible necrotic tissue – a characteristic of the majority of fungating tumours. The malodorous volatile fatty acids that are released as a metabolic end-product are responsible for the characteristic smell and profuse exudate often associated with these wound types – the exudate being attributed to the activity of bacterial enzymes (proteases) and their role in tissue breakdown. Stagnant exudate may also be responsible for any odour in the wound,[1,9] and needs to be considered carefully, and incorporated into, wound assessment criteria.

Identifying the problem

Patients with fungating wounds may present at an early stage with advanced conditions, or only when metastatic disease is evident. This may be recognised by the patient because of the development of unanticipated additional lesions.

Diagnosis is based on histological assessment. Cultures taken from the surface of the wounds usually confirm the presence of anaerobic organisms such as *Bacteroides*. If the presence of these organisms is not dealt with appropriately, the result will be the production of by-products such as propionic, lactic and succinic acids, which if not controlled by the use of appropriate absorbent dressing materials (e.g. alginates) will quickly result in maceration of, and damage to, the tissue surrounding the original lesion.

Key tip 7.3

Maceration may be defined as the stripping/excoriation of the epidermis due to the *prolonged* presence of toxins on the skin.

Identification of these metabolic end-products usually involves gas-liquid chromatography analysis. This is a practical, inexpensive procedure that can be undertaken in the clinical laboratory.

It should be emphasised that the presence of a fungating wound is not necessarily an intractable problem. Therefore, the medical aims of treatment and patient management may be identified in the first instance as:

- control of growth of the tumour
- arresting surface haemorrhage
- if possible, preserving or restoring the viability of the patient's tissues.

Treatment protocols may include one or more of the following:

- radiotherapy
- surgery
- laser therapy
- cytotoxic or hormone replacement therapy

- control of any symptomatology displayed by the patient either during or after treatment.

Key tip 7.4

The effects need to be assessed as part of the holistic patient assessment, addressed sympathetically, and all observations utilised in order to direct appropriate interventions, including those local to the wound (i.e. the use of wound management materials).

A focused assessment – holistic perspective

It is imperative that professionals adopt a holistic approach to the management of the patient and wound – acknowledging the interrelationship between the two – in order to facilitate objective *and* quality-management strategies.

A nursing model (e.g. Activities of Living[10]) aids the identification of the patient's problems and needs, and can be used by all members of the intra- and inter-disciplinary team to plan, structure and implement interventions designed to have a positive impact on the patient's current and future lifestyle.

Maintaining a safe environment

This is important to reduce the risk of infection (either local or systemic), as this may complicate wound assessment *and* the overall patient wound management plan. Wound infection can be the cause of discomfort and may result in odours being associated with the lesion as a result of anaerobic activity, e.g. as with bacteroidal colonisation.

Nearly 100% of all wounds (particularly chronic wounds that have accessible necrotic tissue within their margins) will be colonised by some organism; most commonly the hosts *Staphylococcus aureus*. However, the presence of bacteria or slough within the wound margins alone may not be of any clinical significance.[11]

Key tip 7.5

An infected wound may be defined as one that has been colonised by organisms that have become pathogenic and resulted in an adverse host reaction (e.g. pus production or additional tissue breakdown).

Communication

The importance of communication cannot be overemphasised. This is crucial to the patient and family psychological wellbeing. It is important to keep the patient informed of the:

- general condition

- prognosis
- state of the wound.

Anxiety caused by a lack of information can impair and adversely affect the patient's natural healing potential.[12]

Occasionally the malignant lesion may invade the patient's head and neck region.[13] If this happens the patient's speech may be adversely affected. Therefore, it may be appropriate to encourage the patient to write down all that they would otherwise have spoken.[14] In addition, observation of body language is an important skill in enabling cues to be identified and effectively explored.

Breathing

Breathing techniques ensure adequate ventilation and help to maintain an oxygen-rich supply to the wound, thereby optimising any healing potential.[15] Both progressive disease and the ageing process can alter this practice. The specific evidence for the role of oxygen in wound healing, which can often appear contradictory, has been discussed elsewhere.[15]

Eating and drinking

A balanced dietary intake is important to ensure the provision of essential nutrients such as protein, vitamins (A, B_{12} and C) minerals (zinc and iron) and carbohydrates. If it is not practical for the patient to take oral supplements – because of the side effects of any chosen 'treatment' modality – then the hospital or community nutrition and dietetics department should be contacted and advice sought about an alternative approach to the delivery of the nutrients.

Elimination

Urinary or faecal incontinence may be either a concern or a problem for the patient if the malignant lesion is in the perianal region, or is the cause of a fistula involving either the bladder or the bowel. In many cases, suprapubic urinary catheters will be inserted and colostomies performed electively in order to alleviate the patient's symptomatology.[16]

Maintaining body temperature

Hypothermia can delay the healing process significantly.[17] Any interventions such as the use of cold solutions or leaving the wound exposed for prolonged periods of time (e.g. when another colleague is expected to visit the clinical area to assess or give an opinion on ongoing wound management) should be avoided. Pyrexia may be an indication of wound infection. If an infection is inappropriately treated and the pyrexia is prolonged, for each degree rise in body temperature the metabolic demands of the patient are increased by 10%.[18]

Mobilisation

If mobility of either an individual limb, or the whole body, is reduced, this can result in associated joint stiffness and muscle atrophy inducing circulatory stasis. This may predispose the patient to the development of pressure ulcers[19] or deep vein thrombosis, further complicating the management of the medical condition.

Expressing sexuality

Disfiguring lesions (*see* Figure 7.1) can increase anxiety and sense of isolation because of an altered body image.[20] Often feelings range from embarrassment (*'nobody will want to talk to me'*) through to depression, and may be the sole reason for a change in the patient's lifestyle. Typical reactions and feelings that this group of patients may encounter have been summarised as the *SCARED syndrome* (*see* Table 7.1).[21]

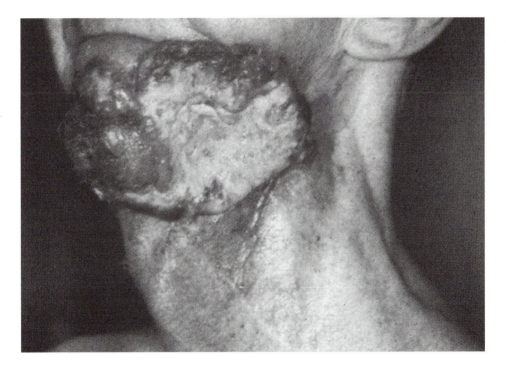

Figure 7.1   Disfiguring lesions. © 2005 Mark Collier.

Table 7.1 The SCARED syndrome[21]

You			They	
Feel	Behave		Behave	Feel
Self-conscious	Submissive	S	Staring	Sympathy
Conspicuous	Clumsy	C	Curious	Caution
Angry	Apathetic	A	Awkward	Anguish
Resentful	Regressive	R	Rude	Reluctance
Empty	Excluded	E	Evasive	Embarrassment
Different	Defenceless	D	Distance	Dread

Psychological issues

When anxiety level is increased, perception of pain related to any wound management techniques can be significantly heightened.[22] In addition, any pain experienced in association with fungating wounds may be increased by the fear of visualising the lesion and further exacerbated by odour and/or the fear of dying.[23]

The main source of malodour related to skin ulcers such as fungating wounds (other than stagnant exudate) are two key impact odours which can trigger a gagging or vomit reflex in patients and carers. This particular malodour is detectable and persistent, thereby increasing the patient's self-consciousness about it, which may inhibit them, for example, from inviting friends to visit.[24]

Dying

The ideal aim of wound healing may be unrealistic in the terminally ill patient, and the choice of dressing materials used may be influenced more by the need to maintain or enhance the patient's quality of life.[25] Therefore, it is essential to explore the patient's choice of care setting at an early stage, especially if the tumour is malignant and the prognosis poor.[26]

Key tip 7.6

Every effort must be made to ensure that the patient achieves as peaceful a death as possible with all relevant support and services available.

Sleeping

Sleep is an essential factor in tissue regeneration. Sleep encourages the release of testosterone, prolactin, somatotrophin and growth hormone.[27] Encourage the patient to rest, especially if s/he is receiving aggressive rather than palliative therapies. Occasionally, mild sedatives and relaxants may be prescribed to facilitate periods of rest.

Diversional therapy

Patients with fungating wounds at all stages of treatment can be encouraged to adopt as normal a lifestyle as possible, continuing to pursue any hobbies and maintain interests such as photography, listening to music, watching television or gentle gardening.

Religion/spirituality

Every effort should be made to explore and meet the identified needs of the individual.

Principles of wound assessment

It is important to consider the specifics of assessment in order to ensure that any planned interventions do not adversely interact with any course of treatment currently being undertaken. Discussion of the principles of wound assessment can be expanded by reading reference 9.

The process of wound assessment should incorporate the:

- professionals' knowledge of relevant anatomy and physiology (including the normal wound-healing process)
- collection of objective and subjective data
- analysis and interpretation of the information obtained
- identification of the patient's problems and needs through discussion
- goal-planning and care regimen.[28,29]

The common symptoms associated with fungating lesions include:

- malodour
- exudate
- pain
- bleeding
- pruritis
- cellulitis.[29]

Common characteristics associated with fungating wounds are that they include the:

- presence of necrotic tissue
- clinical signs of infection.

Specific wound assessment should highlight the characteristics of the wound and the associated symptoms, e.g.

- size
- location
- percentage of devitalised material noted within the wound margins
- amount and nature of any exudate being produced by the wound
- whether any odour can be associated with the lesion
- the nature and type of pain that can be directly attributed to the fungating wound

- the effects on the patient's activities of daily living
- the current state of the surrounding skin immediately adjacent to the wound.[4]

A number of specialist wound assessment guides include the *Teler indicator*[30] and *Wound Symptoms Self Assessment Chart (WoSSAC)*.[31] The latter considers factors such as:

- the effect of the fungating lesion on the patient's relationships within the family
- the ability to socialise generally.

In addition, flow charts (*see* Figure 7.2[32]) can assist the specific assessment process.

Noting wound location aids identification of the cause of the wound, especially in the case of chronic wound types (the classification most relevant to fungating lesions). In addition, it can alert the professional to potential and actual problems that may be experienced by the patient and professional dealing with the lesion. For example:

- for the patient a fungating wound close to the axilla or any joint may impair normal movements thus affecting the normal activities of daily living
- for the professional the location, size and shape of the wound can give rise to considerable challenges in the fitting and securing of dressings[29] which can lead to other difficulties for the patient and professional related to the frequency of, and the pain associated with, dressing changes.[33]

Measuring wound size is important for the minimisation of unwanted syptomatology, as well as for accurate visual records of the change in surface area of an open wound in order to identify any trend associated with the latter. For example:

- is the wound showing signs of improvement?
- is the wound deteriorating?

There are a number of methods available for assessing wounds visually including:

- *computer mapping*
- *Polaroid or digital-type photography* – incorporating a scale such as a paper ruler within the frame near to the wound
- *tracing wounds using a clean transparent film or sheet* – tracing these wound types should be treated with caution; local bleeding from the surface of the wound may be induced as a result of contact between the tracing material and friable tissues.

Wound photography provides a two-dimensional representation of the wound. However, there are difficulties in using the results for comparative purposes as there is a need to ensure that the camera angle, focal length and patient position are consistent.[34,35] Perhaps more importantly, the sensitive position of the wound may preclude the use of this data-collection method in the first instance – that is, until a positive rapport has been established between the professional and patient. In addition, the full extent of the wound may not be seen, as in the case of undermining. In an attempt to combat this, ultrasound imaging has been considered as an assessment tool for fungating wounds.[36] However, this method has been rejected:

> *on the grounds that the intrusion to the patient was not justified relative to the quality of the information obtained.*[36]

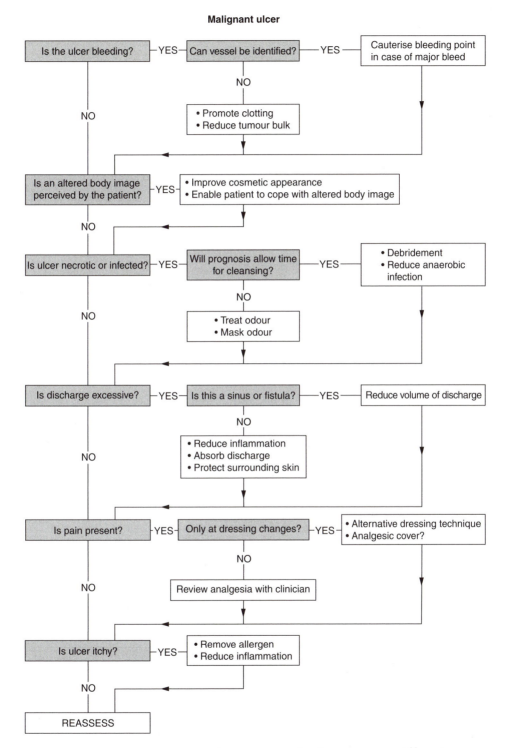

Figure 7.2 Management guidelines for a patient with a fungating wound.[32]

Assessing the wound bed/percentage of devitalised tissue

The use of classification tools *(see* reference 9) is important in order to take into account the amount of tissue destruction noted within the wound margins and to assess the major characteristics of the tissues seen within those margins. Are they:

- necrotic
- sloughy
- granulating?

More recently the concept of wound bed preparation[37] has become associated with the assessment of devitalised tissues within wounds, and the TIME framework, found to be particularly helpful by practitioners for the specific/focused assessment of chronic skin lesions such as fungating wounds, was developed in conjunction with this concept.[38]

TIME framework

- **T** – *Tissues*: what tissue types can be identified within the wound margins?
- **I** – *Inflammation*: are there signs of inflammation and/or clinical infection? If so, what is the anticipated effect on the identified patient outcomes?
- **M** – *Moisture*: not only is the wound bed moist but what are the components of the moisture? Is there anything missing?
- **E** – *Edges*: are the edges of the lesion raised? Are they showing signs of excoriation/maceration?

Assessing wound odour and the skin surrounding the wound

When a fungating wound is assessed the subjective reporting by the patient of the presence of any odour should guide the subsequent treatment regimes. This is important as the professional can become desensitised to odour as a result of repeated exposure to wounds with similar symptomatology.

Key tip 7.7

Malodours associated with fungating wounds usually result from the presence of both aerobic and anaerobic organisms within the wound margins.[1]

The condition of the skin surrounding the wound can indicate the presence of wound infection. The clinical signs include:

- inflammation
- localised erythema
- heat
- pain.

This highlights a problem of tissue excoriation or maceration caused by excessive production of exudate that is inappropriately allowed to remain on the patient's skin. The use of alcohol-free barrier products can provide protection for up to 72 hours before reapplication is required.[39]

Assessing wound pain

Wound pain assessment involves:

- observing the depth of the wound
- noting critical factors such as:
  - the *type of pain* reported
  - its *severity*, *duration* and any *precipitating factors* – e.g. is pain only reported at night when the number of distracters are reduced and the patient has time to focus on his or her body?

Control of pain may be achieved by using appropriate analgesia and a wound dressing that does not adhere to the wound surface.[40] Topical gel analgesia has proved successful.[41] However, be acutely aware of the product licence governing the analgesic being considered.

Assessing wound bleeding

Fungating malignant wounds have fragile surfaces and will often be associated with local bleeding – characteristically a slow ooze. The use of wound contact materials (non-adherent dressing products) and gentle wound irrigation can reduce the risk of wound bleeding.[29]

Additional measures to reduce the risk of bleeding include:[39]

- oral tranexamic acid for up to 10 days
- the use of topical sucralfate paste
- topical adrenaline can be applied to areas that are bleeding heavily to induce local vasoconstriction; however, excessive use may cause tissue necrosis
- haemostatic surgical dressings can be considered for the control of heavier bleeding.

Documentation of wound assessments

Wound assessment can be enhanced by the use of a reliable and systematic chart.[42,43] As a consequence of a systematic wound assessment the following should be asked:

1 What is the aetiology and location of the wound?
2 How should the wound be graded using an 'objective' grading tool?
3 Based on the identified wound grading, what is the primary treatment objective for this wound as seen?
4 What treatment regime is required in order to facilitate the achievement of the identified treatment objective?

The primary goal of *wound healing* may not be appropriate for all patients with fungating wounds. However, treatment objectives identified as a result of the assessment process should include:

- clean/deslough/debride the wound surface
- control and minimise the effects of any wound exudate
- protect the surrounding skin

- minimise the effects of any complications associated with the lesion such as increased bacterial burden/wound infection
- control and minimise the effects of any bleeding associated with the wound
- control and minimise any offensive odour(s)
- control and minimise any associated wound pain
- optimise the local healing environment
- optimise the patient's healing potential.

Principles of wound management

Although the principles of optimum wound management should always be remembered,[15,44] it is the problems *perceived by the patient* that structure the wound management plan.

Wound cleansing

Unless otherwise prescribed, the wound-cleansing agent of choice – if indicated at all – would be normal saline 0.9%. In addition, topical antibacterial agents such as metronidazole gel (otherwise known as Metrotop) may be used in conjunction with appropriate dressing materials[45,46] in order to aid the control of any perceived wound odours as discussed previously.

Wound management

In addition to the wound management treatment objectives previously highlighted, consider the following when choosing a wound-dressing material as part of the management plan for a patient with a fungating wound:[46]

- the control of pain through the maintenance of optimum humidity at the wound site by using dressings that do not adhere to the tumour
- restoration of body symmetry by the use of cavity dressings
- achievement of cosmetic acceptability without the need for bulky secondary dressings.

The following wound management and dressing protocol might be considered (*see* Figure 7.3 – colour plate section):

- *activated charcoal* – odorous lesions[47] but not if heavily exuding
- *alginates (flat/ribbon/packing)* – exuding and/or bleeding wounds[39]
- *foams/hydropolymers* – for exuding wounds and may occasionally be used in conjunction with alginates[48]
- *hydrogel sheets* – for the symptomatic relief of pruritis[31]
- *hydrocolloid sheets* – lightly exuding wounds, or for protection of the surrounding skin[49]
- *semi-permeable film membranes* – for protection only and then only if the surrounding skin is intact; dressings that have a high moisture vapour transfer rate appear to vent excess fluid as opposed to allowing it to accumulate[50]
- *siliconised wound contact materials* – to minimise local trauma at the time of dressing changes[51]

- *topical antimicrobials* – e.g. iodine and silver-based wound-dressing materials may be considered for assisting the wound cleaning process or reducing the bacterial burden on the wound surface or for minimising the effects of local infection – assessed by the presence of clinical signs; however, should any adverse effects be reported by the patient, such as an increase in associated wound pain, then the use of the same should be discontinued
- *secondary dressings of choice* – remembering not to compromise the patient's skin by inappropriate use of adhesive tapes/fixations.

For the primary functions of interactive wound management materials (dressing products identified by generic classification) read references 15 and 44.

Conclusion

As with any wound management scenario, it is important to evaluate interventions at intervals dictated by the *systematic* and *holistic assessment* of patient and the wound.

Caring for the individual with a fungating lesion is challenging *and* rewarding, especially for the professional who is ideally placed to enhance the quality of the care that the patient receives, either as a result of one's own actions, or by identifying the need for other professionals from the intra-/interdisciplinary team, further to one's holistic assessment of the patient.

> *If you keep in mind the patient's best interests you will be their best friend, advocate and carer.*

Self-assessment exercise 7.1
Time: 5 minutes

Highlight or tick the correct answer.

1 Which of the following has been reported to be the most common anatomical site for the development of a fungating wound?
   a Abdomen.
   b Breast.
   c Chest.
   d Digits.
2 The most common symptoms associated with fungating wounds are all listed in which of the following?
   a Malodour, exudate, pain, bleeding, vasculitis and cellulitis.
   b Malodour, exudate, pain, bleeding, pruritis and cellulitis.
   c Malodour, exudate, pain, erythema, pruritis and cellulitis.
   d Malodour, exudate, pain, haemorrhage, pruritis and vasculitis.
3 The principle on which modern wound management interventions are based involves ensuring that the following environment is maintained at the wound interface.
   a Warm and dry.
   b Cold and dry.
   c Warm and moist.
   d Cold and moist.

4 When attempting to measure the size of a fungating lesion, all of the following techniques may be considered except one. Which is it?
   a Computer mapping.
   b Two-dimensional photography.
   c Wound mapping.
   d Ultrasound.

5 All of the following wound management materials have been identified as appropriate for the management of malignant fungating lesions except one. Which is it?
   a Alginates.
   b Foams.
   c Hydrocolloids.
   d Particulates.

6 Wound management protocols and guidelines are useful as they can be best described as?
   a Ensuring that all fungating wounds are covered with the same product.
   b Ensuring that all nurses use wound management materials in the same way for the management of patients with fungating lesions.
   c Ensuring that fungating wounds are covered with the most appropriate wound-dressing materials in order to manage assessed associated symptomatology.
   d Ensuring that only the most expensive evidence-based products are used for the management of patients with fungating wounds.

(*See* answers on page 129.)

Post-reading exercise 7.1
Time: 30 minutes

- Return to the notes that you made during Pre-reading exercise 7.1.
- Reflect in the light of what you have now been introduced to.
- Highlight any changes that you might make to your approach should you have the opportunity to care for a similar patient.
- Discuss your thoughts with your colleague, identifying the rationale that underpins any changes you may have highlighted.

References

1   Neal K. Treating fungating wounds. *Nursing Times*. 1991; **7**: 85–86.
2   Mortimer P. Skin problems in palliative care: medical aspects. In: Doyle D, Hanks C, MacDonald N, editors. *Oxford Textbook of Palliative Medicine*. Oxford: Oxford Medical Publications; 1993.
3   Collier M. The assessment of patients with malignant fungating wounds – an holistic approach. Part one. *Nursing Times*. 1998; **93**: Suppl.
4   Collier M. The holistic management of fungating wounds. *Nursing Notes*. 1997; **14**: 2–5.
5   Ivetic O, Lyric P. Fungating arid ulcerating malignant lesions: a review of the literature. *J Adv Nursing*. 1990; **15**: 83–88.

6   Thomas S. *Current Practices in the Management of Fungating Lesions and Radiation-damaged Skin.* Bridgend: Surgical Materials Testing Laboratory; 1992.

7   Willis R. *The Spread of Tumours in the Human Body,* 3rd edition. London: Butterworths; 1973.

8   Grocott P. The palliative management of fungating malignant wounds. *J Wound Care.* 1995; **4:** 240–242.

9   Collier M. Assessing a wound — RCN Nursing Update (Unit 29). *Nursing Standard.* 1994; **8** (Suppl.): 3–8.

10 Roper N, Logan W, Tierney A. *The Elements of Nursing.* Edinburgh: Churchill Livingstone; 1985.

11 Ayliffe G, Geddes A, Lowburv E *et al. Control of Hospital-acquired Infection.* 3rd edition. London: Chapman and Hall; 1992.

12 Boore J. *Prescription for Recovery.* London: Royal College of Nursing; 1978.

13 McElney M. The psychological effects of head and neck surgery. *J Wound Care.* 1993; **2:** 47–52.

14 Saunders S. Mutual support. Wound care nursing supplement. *Nursing Times.* 1993; **32:** 76–82.

15 Collier M. Principles of optimum wound management. *Nursing Standard.* 1991; **10:** 47–52.

16 Carville K. Caring for cancerous wounds in the community. *J Wound Care.* 1995; **4:** 66–68.

17 Collier M. Wound assessment – making informed choices. *Practice Nursing.* 1990; **November:** 17–18.

18 Moody M. Problem wounds: a nursing challenge – RCN Nursing Update (Unit 17). *Nursing Standard.* 1992; **7**(6): 3–8.

19 Collier M. *Pressure Sore Development and Prevention. Educational leaflet 3.* Huntingdon: Wound Care Society; 1989.

20 Topping A. The trauma of burns. *Wound Management.* 1992; **2:** 8–9.

21 Partridge J. *Changing Faces – the challenge of facial disfigurement.* Harmondsworth: Penguin; 1990.

22 Hargreaves A, Lander J. Use of transcutaneous nerve stimulation for postoperative pain. *Nursing Res.* 1989; **38:** 159–161.

23 Hollinworth H. *Pain. Educational leaflet 4.* Huntingdon: Wound Care Society; 1997.

24 Van Toller S. Invisible wounds: the effects of skin ulcer malodours. *J Wound Cure.* 1994; **3:** 103–105.

25 Franks P. Quality of life as an outcome indicator. In: Morison M, Moffatt C, Bale S *et al.,* editors. *Nursing Management of Chronic Wounds.* London: Mosby; 1997, Chapter 13.

26 Collier M. The assessment of patients with malignant fumigating wounds – an holistic approach. Part two. *Nursing Times.* 1998; **93** (Suppl.): 1–4.

27 Torrance C. Sleep and wound healing. *Surg Nurse.* 1990; **3:** 16–20.

28 Collier M. The elements of wound assessment. *Nursing Times.* 2003; **99**(13): Suppl.

29 Naylor W. Malignant wounds: aetiology and principles of management. *Nursing Standard.* 2002; **16**(52): 45–53.

30 www.teler.com.

31 Naylor W, Laverty D, Mallet J. *The Royal Marsden Hospital Handbook of Wound Management in Cancer Care.* Oxford: Blackwell Scientific; 2001.

32 Saunders J, Regnard C. Management of malignant ulcers – a flow diagram. *Palliative Medicine.* 1989; **3:** 153–155.

33 Bird C. Managing malignant fungating wounds. *Professional Nurse.* 2000; **15**(4): 253–256.

34 Griffen J, Tolley E, Tooms R *et al.* A comparison of photographic and transparency based methods for measuring wound surface area. *Physical Therapy.* 1993; **73:** 117–122.

35 Thomas A, Wysocki A. The healing wound: a comparison of three clinically useful methods of measurement. *Decubitus.* 1991; **3:** 18–25.

36 Grocott P. Assessment of fungating wounds. *J Wound Care.* 1995; **4:** 333–336.

37 Collier M. Wound bed management: key principles for practice. *Professional Nurse.* 2002; **18**(4): 221–225.

38 Dowsett C, Ayello E. TIME principles of chronic wound bed preparation and management. *British Journal of Nursing.* 2004; **13**(15): Suppl. 16–24.

39 McMurray V. Managing patients with fungating malignant wounds. *Nursing Times.* 2003; **99**(13): Suppl.

40 Pudner R. The management of patients with a fungating or malignant wound. *Journal of Community Nursing.* 1998; **12**(9): 30–34.

41 Grocott P. The management of fungating wounds. *Journal of Wound Care*. 1999; **8**(5): 232–234.

42 Morison M. Wound care – a problem solving approach. RCN Nursing Update. *Nursing Standard*. 1992; **37**(6) Suppl: 9–14.

43 Flanagan M. *Wound Management. ACE Series*. Edinburgh: Churchill Livingstone; 1998.

44 Collier M. *Wound Care: Mims for Nurses Pocket Guide*. London: Haymarket Medical Imprint; 2003.

45 Thomas S. *Wound Management and Dressings*. London: Pharmaceutical Press; 1990.

46 Grocott P. Application of the principles of modern wound management for complex wounds. In: *Proceedings of the First European Conference on the Advances of Wound Management*. London: EMAP; 1992.

47 Kelly N. Malodorous fungating wounds: a review of current literature. *Professional Nurse*. 2002; **17**(5): 323–326.

48 Naylor W. Using a new foam dressing in the care of fungating wounds. *British Journal of Nursing*. 2001; **10**(6): S24–30.

49 Thomas S. Assessment and management of wound exudate. *Journal of Wound Care*. 1997; **6**(7): 327–330.

50 Grocott P. Exudate management in fungating wounds. *Journal of Wound Care*. 1998; **8**(5): 232–234 .

51 Hollinworth H, Collier M. Nurses' views about pain and trauma at the time of dressing changes: results of a national survey. *Journal of Wound Care*. 2000; **9**(8): 369–374.

To learn more

- Collier M. *Wound Care: Mims for Nurses Pocket Guide*. London: Haymarket Medical Imprint; 2003.
- Grocott P, Browne N, Cowley S. WRAP: defining clinical needs for fluid handling devices. *Wounds UK*. 2005; **1**(2): 11–16.
- Hack A. Malodorous wounds – taking the patient's perspective into account. *Journal of Wound Care*. 2003; **12**(8): 319–321.
- Wilkes L, Boxer E, White K. The hidden side of nursing: why caring for patients with malignant malodorous wounds is so difficult. *Journal of Wound Care*. 2003; **12**(2): 76–80.

Complementary chapters

See also Stepping into Palliative Care 1: relationships and responses

- Chapter 2: What is palliative care?
- Chapter 3: The cancer journey
- Chapter 4: The experience of illness
- Chapter 5: The psychological impact of serious illness
- Chapter 6: Hope and coping strategies
- Chapter 7: The therapeutic relationship
- Chapter 11: The value of teamwork
- Chapter 13: Communication: the essence of good practice, management and leadership
- Chapter 15: Transcultural and ethnic issues at the end of life
- Chapter 16: Sexuality and palliative care

See also Stepping into Palliative Care 2: care and practice

- Chapter 1: Assessment in palliative care
- Chapter 2: Introduction to pain management
- Chapter 9: The last few days of life
- Chapter 13: Spirituality and palliative care
- Chapter 15: Complementary therapies: a therapeutic model for palliative care

---

Answers to Self-assessment exercise 7.1

1 b.
2 b.
3 c.
4 c.
5 d.
6 c.

Chapter 8

Emergencies in palliative care

Jenny Forrest and Mark Napier

> **Pre-reading exercise 8.1**
> **Time: 10 minutes**
>
> 1 What constitutes a palliative care emergency?
> 2 What questions would you ask when considering management of emergencies in patients with advanced disease?

Introduction

Emergencies in advanced terminal disease are common. They are often stressful for the patient, family and professional. In this chapter, we will look at the recognition and management of common palliative care emergencies. The definition of a palliative care emergency depends on the clinical situation and the event. The onset of signs of spinal cord compression in a patient with slowly progressive prostate cancer requires immediate attention, whereas the same signs in a patient confined to bed, because of general debility from progressive liver metastases, would not.

Before taking action, consider:

- the patient's general condition
- the disease
- the prognosis
- the patient's and family's wishes
- any proposed treatment
- the distress caused by the symptoms.[1]

Some emergencies are predictable from the nature of the disease. Early intervention can lead to effective treatment. If intervention is inappropriate, early discussion with professionals, patient and family may reduce the stress of unexpected developments, and the need for urgent clinical decisions. This must be balanced against the possible increased anxiety that the event will happen (*see* Box 8.1).

Common emergencies to be considered include:

- spinal cord compression
- superior vena cava obstruction
- neutropaenic sepsis
- hypercalcaemia

- tumour lysis syndrome
- haemorrhage.

Box 8.1   Questions to ask when considering management of patients in a palliative care setting

- What is the problem?
- Is it reversible?
- How distressed is the patient by the symptoms?
- What are the patient's wishes?
- What are the family's wishes?
- Would active treatment maintain or improve the patient's quality of life?

Spinal cord compression (SCC)

Malignant spinal cord compression is a common complication of cancer and has a substantial and sudden negative effect on both quality of life and survival. It is important to identify early and act quickly.

Self-assessment exercise 8.1
Time: 10 minutes

- What are the commonest cancers causing spinal cord compression (SCC)?
- What are the signs and symptoms of SCC?

Almost any systemic cancer can metastasise to the spinal column and cause SCC (*see* Box 8.2). However, the more common the cancer, the more likely it will spread to the vertebral column and cause SCC.

Patients can present with SCC as the first symptom of cancer (*see* Figure 8.1). SCC is usually caused by extradural metastasis but it can arise from intradural metastasis. Cord damage arises from extension of a vertebral body metastasis into the epidural space in 85% of cases. Alternative mechanisms include:

- vertebral collapse
- direct spread of tumour through the intervertebral foramen
- interruption of the vascular supply.

Treatment aims to reverse the compression prior to the onset of ischaemia and permanent damage.[2]

Box 8.2   Cancers commonly causing spinal cord compression in adults[1]

- *Most common cancer*:
  - prostate
  - breast
  - lung.
- *Common cancer*:
  - non-Hodgkin lymphoma
  - multiple myeloma
  - renal.
- *Less common cancer*:
  - colorectal
  - unknown primary
  - sarcomas.

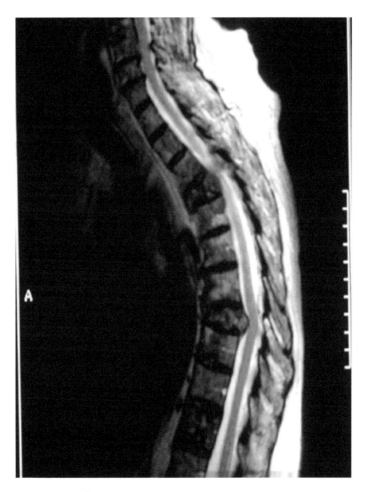

Figure 8.1   Spinal cord compression.

Self-assessment exercise 8.2
Time: 20 minutes

Case scenario 8.1

Sonya (36) was diagnosed with locally advanced breast cancer 3 years ago. This was treated initially with mastectomy, chemotherapy and hormones (zoladex and tamoxifen). Two years later, she presented with hip pain and a bone scan revealed multiple bone metastases. Her tamoxifen was switched to anastrazole. A few months later she attended her general practitioner complaining of a 2-week history of increasing back pain and some weakness in her leg.

Questions:

- How would you assess Sonya?
- What further questions would you ask?
- What would you look for on examination?
- What other factors might you consider?
- If you suspected spinal cord compression what would you do next?
- What is the most important predictor of function after treatment?

Sonia was referred to the local oncology centre where an MRI confirmed SCC and she was treated with steroids and radiotherapy (*see* Figure 8.1). She remained ambulatory and was discharged 1 week later. Ten months later, she re-presented with further leg weakness and became paraplegic. She was again treated with steroids and radiotherapy. She spent 2 months being rehabilitated before returning home walking with a Zimmer frame. A care plan was organised.

Clinical features

Localisation

SCC affects:

- the thoracic spine $(60–80\%)^2$
- the lumbar spine (15–30%)
- the cervical spine (< 10%).

Key tip 8.1

Less than 50% of patients have more than one area of spine affected.[1]

Signs and symptoms

It is important to question and look for the following features:

- *Pain* – 90% of patients have pain at the time of diagnosis for an average of 8 weeks or longer:[2]
  - there is sometimes associated root irritation, causing a band-like pain that is worse on coughing and straining.
- *Motor impairment* – 60–85% of patients have weakness at the time of diagnosis; the most apparent and troublesome symptom:
  - a feeling of 'stiffness' in the legs may herald weakness
  - 66% of patients are unable to walk when they are diagnosed[3]
  - the strongest predictor of response to treatment is the functional status at the time of treatment
  - the majority of those who were able to walk without help retained that ability
  - only a small proportion of paraplegic patients regained mobility or bladder function.

This highlights the need for diagnosis *before* the onset of weakness.[4]

- *Sensory deficits* – patients can be less aware of sensory problems than they are of weakness:
  - beware of the patient with back pain complaining of *'walking on cotton wool'* as an early presentation of SCC
  - tingling and numbness usually starts in both feet and ascends the legs
  - when examining patients for a sensory level ask about altered sensation rather than just loss of sensation
  - when applying light touch to upper chest and comparing it with lower parts of body ask:
    - can you feel this?
    - does it feel the same as this?
  - when applying light touches, moving from an area of decreased sensation to normal sensation ask:
    - where does it change?
- *Bowel and bladder dysfunction* – these tend to occur late and are associated with significant weakness.

Key tip 8.2

Suspect SCC if any of the following present:

- back pain:
  - worse on lying, coughing or straining
  - with radiation
- any sensory change, motor weakness, or sphincter disturbance.

What to do if you suspect SCC

Speed of diagnosis is essential to enable the best outcome. In a patient with known bone metastases, presenting with increasing back pain, and any abnormal neurology, make an emergency referral to the oncologist.

Key tip 8.3

- Early signs are often subtle and easily overlooked – early referral is *important*.
- If you have a suspicion of impending SCC, make *emergency* contact with the oncology centre on-call service to arrange definitive investigation and management.
- *Early diagnosis* improves outcome.

What happens to the patient on admission to hospital?

SCC diagnosis

Clinically suspected SCC must be confirmed by imaging, not only to define the diagnosis, but also to make informed decisions about surgery, radiotherapy, chemotherapy or supportive care and palliation. Involve the multidisciplinary team at the outset, e.g.:

- oncologists
- neurosurgeons
- radiologists
- nurses
- physiotherapists
- occupational therapists.

The imaging method of choice in the assessment of SCC is MRI (*magnetic resonance imaging – see* Figure 8.1). MRI:

- is non-invasive
- has high soft-tissue resolution
- images in several planes
- reconstructs.

Because of the frequency of several levels of compression, imaging of the entire spine is recommended.[2] Where MRI is not available or contraindicated computerised tomography (CT) scanning and myelography can be used. There is little role for bone scanning in the acute setting but if a patient has a normal plain film and bone scan, then the chances of SCC are very low.

Management of suspected SCC

Decisions on investigations performed and treatment depend on:

- the patient's wishes
- stage of disease

- co-morbidity
- prognosis
- signs and symptoms.

On admission, clinically assess patients, as above. If SCC is suspected, then arrange an *urgent MRI*.

- *Corticosteroids* – high doses can improve outcome and are routinely given to patients with SCC.
  - The exact dose remains controversial (consult local guidelines). Usually, 10–20 mg of dexamethasone or equivalent – although doses up to 100 mg have been used.[5]
  - Prophylactic proton pump inhibitors are also used – these protect the stomach from ulceration and help with symptoms of dyspepsia, caused by high dose steroids.
  - If the patient is immobile, consider thrombo-embolic prophylaxis.
- *Radiotherapy* – although the presence of metastatic disease in the spine makes all treatment palliative, reversal of SCC is invaluable in restoring quality of life.
  - Radiotherapy is usually given by conventional external beams.
  - The patient lies either prone or supine and high energy X-rays are focused on the spine.
  - There is no consensus as to the optimum dose.[2,5] Most radiation oncologists use 20–30 Gy in 5–10 fractions.
  - Radiotherapy for SCC has minimal side effects.
  - Mucositis, nausea, dysphagia and diarrhoea may occur when large portions of the gastrointestinal tract are irradiated.
- *Surgery* – surgery remains the only method that leads to immediate relief of SCC and direct mechanical stabilisation of a diseased and weakened vertebral column. Surgery should be considered in the following:
  - any patient with SCC who can undergo decompression and fixation, i.e. there is sufficient non-diseased spine to allow surgical fixation and they are fit enough
  - direct compression in the setting of intraspinal bony fragments
  - an unstable spine
  - impending sphincteric dysfunction that prompts rapid decompression
  - no response to radiotherapy
  - previous radiotherapy to spinal cord tolerance.[2]
- *Physiotherapy, occupational therapy, social services* – physiotherapy, occupational therapy and other social and support services are important in rehabilitating these often severely disabled patients.

Superior vena cava obstruction (SVCO)

Self-assessment exercise 8.3
Time: 15 minutes

Questions:

- What are the signs and symptoms of SVCO?
- What are the causes of SVCO?
- What are the options for management of SVCO?

Case scenario 8.2 (part 1)

Mrs Browne (66), a retired teacher, smoked over 20 cigarettes a day for 51 years. She attended her GP complaining of increasing shortness of breath. Mrs Brown was assessed and admitted to hospital. On arrival, she was breathless at rest. She had mild facial swelling and some dilated veins across her chest wall. Chest X-ray revealed a widened mediastinum.

What is SVCO?

Superior vena cava obstruction (SVCO) results from the compression of the superior vena cava either by a tumour arising in the right main or upper lobe bronchus or by large volume mediastinal lymphadenopathy. Thrombus is a common complication of SVCO.

Clinical features

- *Cardinal features:*
  - face and neck swelling, particularly periorbital oedema
  - non-pulsatile distension of neck veins
  - dilated superficial veins upper chest
  - oedema of hands and arms.
- *Other features:*
  - shortness of breath and tachypnoea
  - cyanosis
  - hoarse voice (probably related to the underlying cause rather than the SVCO *per se*)
  - headache, worse on stooping
  - visual disturbance
  - dizziness and syncope.

What are the common causes of SVCO?

- Primary bronchial carcinoma (65–80%) – non-small cell and small cell.
- Lymphoma (2–10%).
- Other cancers.
- Non-malignant causes (rare, e.g. benign goitre).

Key tip 8.4

SVCO often occurs prior to a diagnosis of cancer and is the presenting symptom.

Management

Admit patients with suspected SVCO to hospital for urgent assessment. In the past, SVCO has been considered a medical emergency. However, for the majority of patients this is no longer thought to be the case. As this is commonly a presenting symptom, it is important to establish an accurate diagnosis with further imaging and histology.[6]

Depending on histology, staging and local expertise, definitive treatment could be:

- *chemotherapy* – especially of small cell lung cancer or lymphoma
- *radiotherapy* – especially non-small cell lung cancer
- *vascular stenting* – should be considered in all cases (*see* Figure 8.2); it can lead to rapid relief of symptoms[6,7]
- *steroids* – are used in addition to radiotherapy to reduce oedema and improve symptoms more quickly.

Case scenario 8.2 (part 2)

Mrs Browne had a CT scan and bronchoscopy. She was found to have non-small cell lung cancer (NSCLC) and was treated with a stent insertion (*see* Figure 8.2) followed by chemotherapy. Prior to stent insertion, an angiogram showed a clot in the superior vena cava. In addition, she received thrombolysis.

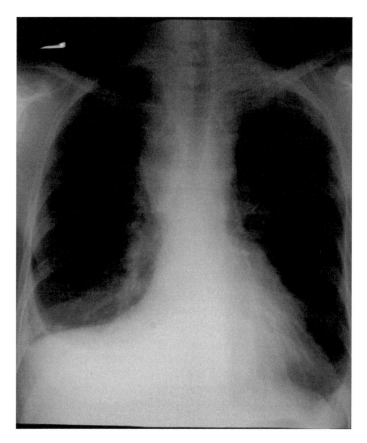

Figure 8.2 Superior vena cava obstruction (SVCO).

Effective anti-cancer therapy in small cell lung cancer, NSCLC and lymphoma improves survival and maintains quality of life. Chemotherapy and/or radiotherapy form the basis of treatment. In small cell lung cancer, stenting is used for relapse of SVCO or persistent SVCO following initial chemotherapy and radiotherapy. In NSCLC, stenting is used for relapsed or persistent SVCO following initial therapy, as well as initial therapy.

Key tip 8.5

In a patient with dyspnoea – *think:*

- SVCO
- *urgent assessment.*

Prognosis

The prognosis of superior vena cava obstruction depends on the underlying condition. In itself, it is not a poor prognostic factor.

Neutropaenic sepsis

Neutropaenic sepsis is a major hazard and the principal cause of treatment-related death associated with the use of cancer chemotherapy. However, if promptly identified and aggressively treated, most episodes can be successfully controlled.[8]

Self-assessment exercise 8.4
Time: 10 minutes

Case scenario 8.3 (part 1)

Mr Smith (57) has a history of colitis. He was recently diagnosed with testicular cancer (teratoma) that had spread to his para-aortic lymph nodes. He commenced on high dose chemotherapy with curative intent. Seven days later, he contacted his GP, complaining of fatigue, shivers, and diarrhoea.

Questions:
You are his doctor.

- What are your concerns?
- What do you do?

Aetiology

Most chemotherapy regimes are toxic to the bone marrow, putting patients at risk of neutropaenia. Life-threatening infection is likely to occur when the total neutrophil count falls below 1.0×10^9/l. The time of highest risk depends on the schedule but is usually 1 to 2 weeks after chemotherapy. The major cause of infection is from host organisms in the bowel or skin. The presence of a central venous line is a further risk.

Clinical features

- *Symptoms*:
  - non-specific symptoms, e.g. fevers, rigors, chills, malaise and anorexia
  - specific symptoms related to site of infection.
- *Signs* – any fever over 38.5°C in a patient with a neutrophil count less than $1.0 \times 10^9/l$ should be considered as systemic infection, even in the absence of any other positive findings:
  - assess for signs of shock: tachycardia, hypotension:
  - look for localising of infection site: chest, urine, line.

Case scenario 8.3 (part 2)

Mr Smith was admitted to hospital. A full blood count showed he was severely neutropaenic (neutrophil count $0.0 \times 10^9/l$). He was dehydrated and septic. Intravenous fluids and antibiotics were administered. Despite this, his condition deteriorated and he was transferred to the intensive care unit. He made a full recovery.

Investigations

Any patient at risk of neutropaenia and found to be febrile requires an urgent blood count. If a low count is confirmed, blood cultures, mid-stream urine for microscopy and culture, throat swab and chest X-ray are required.

Treatment

Broad-spectrum intravenous antibiotics should be urgently instigated. Do not wait for the results of cultures as life-threatening septicaemia may develop.

Neutropaenic patients can deteriorate rapidly. Timely intervention is essential. The condition can be fatal. Mr Smith had a potentially curative tumour, and with the help of the intensivists, he was successfully treated.

All oncology units have guidelines to aid in the diagnosis and rapid treatment of patients with possible/probable neutropaenic sepsis.[9] These stipulate the preferred antibiotic regimens taking into account the local bacterial flora.

Key tip 8.6

All patients on chemotherapy, with a temperature, need an urgent full blood count. If neutropaenic, admit to hospital for blood cultures and intravenous antibiotics. It is appropriate to admit for full assessment and bloods at presentation of pyrexia.

Hypercalcaemia

Self-assessment exercise 8.5
Time: 10 minutes

Case scenario 8.4

Mr Adams (64) presents to the accident and emergency department with confusion and dehydration. The serum calcium is 4.2 mmol/l. He has postural hypotension. On examination, his jugular venous pulse has reduced central venous pressure. He had previously received chemo-radiotherapy for oeso-phageal carcinoma.

Questions:

• How should he be treated?
• What factors will affect your management of him?

Malignant hypercalcaemia is the most common cause of a raised serum calcium. It is the commonest life-threatening metabolic disorder in cancer patients.[1] It has been reported in up to 20–30% of cancer patients at some time during the course of the disease. The detection of hypercalcaemia in cancer patients signifies a poor prognosis. Approximately 50% of patients die within 30 days.[10] However, if the underlying cancer can be treated, survival is extended.

Either of two mechanisms usually cause hypercalcaemia associated with malignancy:

1 local osteolytic hypercalcaemia (20%):
– occurs in patients with bone metastasis
– hypercalcaemia is secondary to increased bone resorption
2 humoral hypercalcaemia of malignancy (80%):
– caused by secretion of parathyroid hormone related protein from cancers.

The tumours that commonly cause this are listed in Table 8.1. However, any tumour can be causative.

Table 8.1 Causes of hypercalcaemia associated with malignancy

Type	Typical tumours
Local osteolytic hypercalcaemia	Breast cancer Multiple myeloma Lymphoma
Humoral hypercalcaemia of malignancy	Squamous-cell cancer, e.g. head and neck, oesophagus, cervix, lung Renal cancer Ovarian cancer Endometrial cancer Breast cancer

---

Key tip 8.7

Most patients have disseminated metastatic disease.

Clinical features

- Weakness.
- Aching.
- Nausea and vomiting.
- Confusion and coma.
- Polyuria and thirst.
- Constipation.
- Anorexia.
- Cardiac arrhythmias.
- Abnormal neurology.
- Dehydration.
- Drowsiness.

Differential diagnosis – other conditions that may present in a similar way to hypercalcaemia

- Diabetes mellitus.
- Cerebral metastases.
- Hepatic or renal failure.
- Neutropaenic sepsis.

Self-assessment exercise 8.6
Time: 5 minutes

- Does hypercalcaemia always need treating?
- If not, when would you treat/not treat?

Investigations

Diagnosis is made on a corrected calcium of more than 2.6 mmol/l. A corrected calcium refers to the measure level being adjusted for the level of albumin in the blood. This is done by the laboratory.

Mild hypercalcaemia is defined as a corrected calcium between 2.7 mmol/l and 3.00 mmol/l. It is often asymptomatic; treatment is only needed if a patient has symptoms.[1]

Self-assessment exercise 8.7

Time: 5 minutes
What factors do you consider, other than the blood calcium level, when deciding how to manage a patient with hypercalcaemia?

Assessment

When deciding on treatment, antihypercalcaemia therapy should be considered as an interim measure with no ultimate effect on survival.[10] Therefore, it is important that the availability of antitumour therapy be considered.

When all available therapies have failed, withholding antihypercalcaemia therapy (which will eventually cause coma and death) may be an appropriate and humane approach. However, for moderate or severe hypercalcaemia, treatment can improve symptoms even in a patient with advanced disease and limited life expectancy. The symptoms experienced depend on the actual level *and* on other factors:

- rate of rise of hypercalcaemia
- age of patient
- other medication, e.g. sedatives or opiates.

The best treatment is tailored to the degree of hypercalcaemia *and* the underlying cause.

Management of hypercalcaemia

- *General supportive measure*:
  - Stop any calcium supplements – as this will augment the hypercalcaemia.
  - Stop medications that may cause hypercalcaemia, e.g. lithium, calcitrol, vitamin D, thiazide diuretics.
  - Discontinue sedative drugs where possible, to reduce neurological symptoms.
  - Promote weight-bearing walking – this helps to stimulate calcium resorption into bones.
  - Replace phosphorous as necessary by oral supplementation – phosphorous is often excreted with calcium by the kidneys.
- *Check bloods* – to monitor the effects of treatment, and dehydration:
  - serum calcium
  - albumin
  - urea
  - electrolytes
  - creatinine.
- *Rehydrate with intravenous fluids* – patients are often dehydrated resulting from a reduction in renal-water-concentrating ability (nephrogenic diabetes insipidus) induced by hypercalcaemia *and* by decreased oral intake (secondary to anorexia, nausea and vomiting):
  - rehydrate with intravenous (IV) fluids (0.9% saline)
  - amount and rate depends on clinical and cardiovascular status, neurological impairment and severity of hypercalcaemia
  - aim to increase the glomerular filtration rate and reduce absorption of calcium by the kidney.
- *Loop diuretics* – diuretics that work on the loop of Henle in the kidney:
  - once the patient is adequately hydrated, loop diuretics can be used to increase renal excretion of calcium.[10]

- *Bisphosphonates* – intravenous bisphosphonates are safe and effective agents for patients with hypercalcaemia associated with malignancy. They work by blocking osteoclastic bone resorption. Two drugs commonly used are:
  - intravenous disodium pamidronate: 60 mg if calcium < 3.0 mmol/l; 90 mg if calcium > 3.0 mmol/l in 500 ml N Saline over 60–90 minutes
  - zoledronic acid 4 mg in 100 ml normal saline over 15 minutes.

  Often regular infusions of bisphosphonates are necessary depending on the availability of other tumour treatments. Before instigating treatment and arranging admission, the patient's wishes, prognosis and general condition should be considered – *is this a terminal event or the first presentation?*
- *Corticosteroids* – useful in haematological malignancies and breast cancer but are rarely used since the availability of intravenous bisphosphonates.

Key tip 8.8

Treatment of hypercalcaemia involves intravenous fluid and intravenous bisphosphonates.

Tumour lysis syndrome

Tumour lysis syndrome comprises a number of metabolic abnormalities that occur as a result of spontaneous or treatment-related cell death. This syndrome arises as a result of rapid breakdown of large numbers of cells, usually at the start of chemotherapy for a highly sensitive tumour, e.g. lymphoma or leukaemia. It leads to extensive metabolic disturbances characterised by hyperkalaemia (raised potassium), hyperuricaemia (raised uric acid), hyperphosphataemia (raised phosphate) and hypocalcaemia (low calcium). In addition, these metabolic upsets can cause renal failure.

Allopurinol is often given, along with adequate hydration to try to prevent the development of tumour lysis syndrome.

Clinical features

- *Hyperkalaemia:*
  - paraesthesias – abnormal feelings of sensation
  - weakness
  - gastrointestinal disturbances
  - arrhythmias
  - cardiac arrest
  - ECG changes – peaked T waves, lengthening PR interval.
- *Hyperuricaemia:*
  - lethargy
  - nausea
  - vomiting.
- *Hyperphosphataemia:*
  - leads to hypocalcaemia.

- *Hypocalcaemia:*
  - spasm
  - convulsions
  - ECG changes – prolonged QT interval.
- *Acute renal failure:*
  - reduced/no urine output
  - swelling
  - hypertension – raised blood pressure.

Management

The best way to reduce the morbidity and mortality of tumour lysis syndrome is to anticipate and prevent it. This is done by the hospital team, as discussed above, by hydration and reduction in uric acid using drugs such as allopurinol. The allopurinol is usually started prior to the chemotherapy and continues for 3 to 4 weeks. It should be noted that it does not need to be continued long term.

If tumour lysis syndrome is suspected, the patient needs *emergency admission* to hospital for blood tests and correction of the metabolic upset. In severe cases, the patient may need haemodialysis.[11]

Haemorrhage

There are many reasons why a patient with cancer may suffer a serious, even life-threatening haemorrhage (*see* Box 8.3).

Box 8.3   Causes of haemorrhage

Several risk factors may co-exist.

- Thrombocytopaenia – low platelets, produced by the bone marrow, important for clotting:
  - *underproduction:*
    - bone marrow infiltration by cancer or leukaemia
    - bone marrow suppression by chemotherapy
  - *increased consumption or destruction:*
    - sepsis or fever.
- Coagulopathy:
  - *disseminated intravascular coagulopathy (DIC):*
    - secondary to infection
    - secondary to cancer/leukaemia
  - *decreased production of coagulation factors:*
    - liver failure
    - vitamin K deficiency.
- Mechanical/vascular factors:
  - *erosion of blood vessels by tumour*
  - *complication of central venous lines.*[11]

In managing the haemorrhage, it is important to consider the

- patient's general condition
- prognosis
- patient's wishes
- underlying cause(s)

when considering treatment options. A patient with advanced cancer, with limited prognosis, may be best managed at home with a syringe driver. However, a patient having potentially curative chemotherapy requires *emergency admission* and it may be appropriate to admit to intensive care or perform emergency surgery.

Management

Management depends not only on the cause, but on other patient factors. If treatment is thought appropriate, then the patient will require *emergency admission* to hospital. In hospital, the acute haemorrhage can, in most cases, be controlled in the short term with:

- appropriate transfusion of platelets or
- coagulation factors plus
- attempts at local haemostasis – direct pressure onto site of bleeding or the packing of the bleeding cavity.

Following this, more definitive treatment will be required to correct the underlying causes, e.g. radiotherapy to a lung cancer that has eroded into a vein to acute haemoptysis – coughing up blood.

Conclusion

In this chapter we have discussed the common oncological emergencies. We have seen how the active management of most emergencies requires emergency admission to hospital.

The fundamental points are:

1 Remember the signs and symptoms of oncological emergencies when assessing a patient with known or suspected cancer.
2 Just because a patient has cancer, it does not mean they should not receive emergency treatment. However, active management is not always in the best interest of the patient.
3 When assessing a patient with cancer it is important to take an holistic approach and ask the following:
   - What do I think is/may be causing their symptoms?
   - What is the patient's general condition?
   - What are the patient's and family's wishes?
   - What is the prognosis?
   - What treatment is available? What does it involve?
   - How much is the patient distressed by their symptoms?
   - What will happen if I do/do not arrange emergency admission?

References

1   Falk S, Fallon M. ABC of palliative care: emergencies. *BMJ*. 1997; **315**: 1525–1528.
2   Prasad D, Schiff D. Malignant spinal cord compression. *The Lancet Oncology*. 2005; **6**(1): 15–24.
3   Husband DJ. Malignant spinal cord compression: prospective study of delays in referral and treatment. *BMJ*. 1998; **317**: 18–21.
4   Baines MJ. Spinal cord compression: a personal and palliative care perspective. *Clinical Oncology*. 2002; **14**:135–138.
5   Loblaw A, Perry J, Chambers A *et al*. Systemic review of the diagnosis and management of malignant extradural spinal cord compression: the cancer care Ontario practice guidelines initiative's neuro-oncology disease site group. *Clinical Oncology*. 2005; **23**(9): 2028–2036.
6   Rowell NP, Gleeson FV. Steroids, radiotherapy, chemotherapy and stents for superior vena caval obstruction in carcinoma of the bronchus: a systemic review. *Clinical Oncology*. 2002; **14**: 338–351.
7   Wilson E, Lyn E, Lynn A *et al*. Radiological stenting provides effective palliation in malignant central venous obstruction. *Clinical Oncology*. 2004; **14**: 228–232.
8   Neal A, Hoskin P. *Clinical Oncology Basic Principles and Practice*. London: Arnold; 2003.
9   Department of Health. *Manual for Cancer Services*. London: Department of Health Publications; 2004.
10 Andrew F, Stewart MD. Hypercalcaemia associated with cancer. *New England Journal of Medicine*. 2004; **352**(4): 373–379.
11 Nicolin G. Emergencies and their management. *European Journal of Cancer*. 2002; **38**: 1365–1377.

To learn more

* Andrew F, Stewart MD. Hypercalcaemia associated with cancer. *New England Journal of Medicine*. 2005; **352**(4): 373–379.
* Prasad D, Schiff D. Malignant spinal cord compression. *The Lancet Oncology*. 2005; **6**(1): 15–24.
* Rowell NP, Gleeson FV. Steroids, radiotherapy, chemotherapy and stents for superior vena caval obstruction in carcinoma of the bronchus: a systemic review. *Clinical Oncology*. 2002; **14**: 338–351.

Complementary chapters

See also Stepping into Palliative Care 1: relationships and responses

* Chapter 3: The cancer journey
* Chapter 4: The experience of illness
* Chapter 5: The psychological impact of serious illness
* Chapter 6: Hope and coping strategies
* Chapter 11: The value of teamwork
* Chapter 14: Ethical dilemmas
* Chapter 15: Transcultural and ethnic issues at the end of life

See also Stepping into Palliative Care 2: care and practice

* Chapter 1: Assessment in palliative care
* Chapter 2: Introduction to pain management
* Chapter 3: Symptom management: a framework
* Chapter 11: Breaking bad news

Chapter 9

The last few days of life

James Gilbert

Pre-reading exercise 9.1
Time: 10 minutes

- Think about how you recognised approaching death in a patient.
- Compare your answers with those at the end of the chapter.

(*See* answers on page 156.)

Introduction

In a book designed to be a practical guide it is important to recognise that the last few days of life can only be identified, with certainty, in retrospect. None the less, for people whose health is deteriorating because of chronic disease – *those requiring palliative care, rather than acute care* – there are established criteria for recognising when death is likely to be imminent.[1] The Liverpool Integrated Care Pathway for the Dying Patient (*discussed in Stepping into Palliative Care 1*) lists four criteria. The patient is:

- bedbound
- semi-comatose
- no longer able to take tablets
- able to take only sips of fluid.

In addition to two of these criteria applying, the clinical team need to agree that there is no realistic reversible cause for the patient's deteriorating health. Importantly, such reversible causes might include:

- metabolic complications, e.g. hypercalcaemia
- the effect of potentially steroid-responsive raised intracranial pressure
- inappropriate drug therapy.

Having mentioned such possibilities, it is important to acknowledge that certainty is rarely achievable anywhere in healthcare. It is especially important in late-stage disease that careful clinical judgement be exercised if people are to be spared burdensome investigations and treatment in the pursuit of certainty.

Overall goals of healthcare

The attempt to prolong life is such a valued and welcomed goal for so much of healthcare that it is unsurprising that many professionals are inclined to pursue life prolongation, at times uncritically. The overall goal of healthcare, to benefit people, is sometimes best achieved by concentrating on helping people die in the best way rather than merely delaying the time of death for as long as possible. This chapter examines how the best help can be provided for those who seem to be in their *last few days of life*.

Physical care

No apology is made for turning first to the physical aspects of care in the last few days of life. Although skilled communication can allay fears, provide emotional support and meet spiritual and social needs, none of these aspects of care are likely to be successful for a patient with serious unrelieved symptoms.

Nursing care

For the majority of people approaching the end of life, it is skilled nursing care that makes the greatest contribution to physical comfort. Specifically, ways of minimising disturbance can be key. The use of modern flotation mattresses has massively reduced the incidence of pressure sores and the need for regular turning of debilitated patients. Bladder catheterisation and external urine drainage devices spare people from the discomfort of toileting, and hoists and sliding sheets allow necessary movements while minimising discomfort. Mouth care, and more specialised nursing techniques of stoma care, tracheostomy management and wound care, have a similarly important role to play.

Drug treatments

While drug therapy makes an important contribution to physical comfort, arguably the most important message is to first *minimise harm caused by drugs* in the last days of life. Many drug treatments can and should be discontinued in late-stage progressive disease.[2] Specifically drugs which become dangerous include:

- *warfarin* – when bleeding becomes more of a risk than embolic disease
- *hypoglycaemic agents* – in particular, metformin – in the face of deteriorating liver and kidney function and diminished nutritional intake
- *diuretics and antihypertensive medication* – frequently become counterproductive, and many drugs are simply unnecessary and burdensome for the patient to take
- *steroids* – discontinuation at the point when they are burdensome to swallow can be safe in late-stage disease when a bedbound patient will not suffer from hypotension, and not benefit from prolonging their dying. The anticonvulsant action of midazolam can be reassuring when steroids are stopped in someone with intracerebral disease.

As with other aspects of care, involving the patient and immediate carers in the decision to discontinue medication is crucial (*see* 'Communication issues' below). The following physical symptoms potentially remediable by drug therapy in the last few days of life include:[3]

- pain
- shortness of breath
- nausea and vomiting
- agitation
- noisy breathing.

Pain

Because of its widespread effectiveness and ease of administration subcutaneously in small volume infusions or injections, *diamorphine* is the mainstay of analgesic treatments. Anti-inflammatory analgesics, such as *diclofenac,* by suppository or the more potent – and more toxic – subcutaneous *ketorolac* also have a part to play. When diamorphine is unavailable *morphine* is equally effective though less easy to administer in very high dosage. Transdermal analgesics such as *fentanyl* and *buprenorphine* are difficult to titrate against variable pain and are therefore less suitable in late-stage disease. However, when analgesic requirements are stable there is no necessity to switch to the subcutaneous route. For a patient using transdermal analgesia successfully, who requires round the clock pain relief, *morphine* or *diamorphine* can be added to a subcutaneous infusion to increase the total opioid dose by *20 to 25%* while continuing the transdermal patch. Such practice avoids the difficulties of delayed and unpredictable reduction in opioid effect following removal of an analgesic patch.

Shortness of breath

In late-stage disease, and when interventions to improve gas exchange are not feasible, feelings of breathlessness and associated panic can be effectively ameliorated by *opioids* and *benzodiazepines*. Specifically sublingual *lorazepam* 0.5 mg to 1 mg or subcutaneous *midazolam* 5–10 mg can be effective, not only in anxiety and as a relaxant but also in reducing sensations of shortness of breath. *Opioids* have also been shown to reduce breathlessness without improving gas exchange[4] and doses above *diamorphine* 10–20 mg (morphine 15–30 mg) subcutaneously are rarely required. Although antibiotics are rarely indicated in late-stage disease, they can on occasion reduce sputum production usefully. Oxygen is rarely indicated and can result in unintended restriction of mobility but nebulised saline can help in moistening and loosening tenacious secretions.

Nausea and vomiting

As oral intake declines in late-stage disease, nausea and vomiting often become less of a problem. However, *levomepromazine* or *haloperidol* are helpful for nausea of chemical causes, e.g.

- renal failure
- hypercalcaemia
- other less readily measurable toxins.

Metoclopramide subcutaneously or *domperidone* rectally can be effective in gastric stasis and intestinal paresis. Propulsive agents such as metoclopromide and domperidone are to be avoided in established intestinal obstruction for fear of worsening colic or risking intestinal perforation. *Cyclizine* is indicated for vomiting of central cause associated with cerebral metastatic disease or inner ear/vestibular problems in which nystagmus can be a helpful clinical sign.

Agitation and restlessness

Most agitation and restlessness in late-stage disease has no realistically reversible cause. Therefore, symptomatic treatment is required. The two commonly useful agents are *midazolam* and *levomepromazine*. Midazolam is to be favoured where anxiety or muscle twitching is prominent and has anticonvulsant action useful in patients with cerebral metastatic disease in whom steroid treatment may recently have been stopped. However, midazolam is not effective against hallucinations, paranoia or other forms of thought disorder. Major tranquillisers such as levomepromazine or haloperidol may be useful in combination with *midazolam* in late-stage restlessness and agitation associated with such thought disorder.

Noisy breathing

Profound weakness in the last few days of life can result in an inability to clear normal respiratory secretions with the result that breathing becomes noisy – sometimes referred to as 'death rattle'. Antimuscarinic agents can reduce the volume of respiratory, and other, secretions although this is sometimes at the expense of making such secretions thicker and more tenacious. *Hyoscine hydrobromide* has useful antisecretory properties in this situation in a dosage of 400–600 micrograms prn or 1.2–2.4 mg subcutaneously over 24 hours. Central sedation is an important, though not always unwelcome, side effect. *Glycopyrrolate* is an alternative less-sedating agent.

Communication issues

In addition to the careful and unhurried identification and exploration of the patient's concerns, much of which will have been done well before the last few days of life, efforts need to be directed at assessing, and providing for, the needs of those close to the person dying. In this respect, use of the term 'relatives' should be taken to include not only those related genetically and by marriage, but partners, whether of the same or different sex, and close friends. Lengthy conversations may not always be necessary particularly where the offer to talk is spontaneous rather than just responsive. The feeling among relatives that their needs are unimportant is both common and wrong. Successfully caring for the dying is very challenging. It is in the dying person's interests that the relatives are well supported in this activity. The medium- to long-term psychological health of the bereaved is improved by identifying satisfactorily their concerns. Commons concerns for relatives include:[3]

- the patient's diminishing food and fluid intake

- the patient's distressing symptoms (confusion, cognitive failure, noisy breathing)
- the patient falling or dying at home
- how the patient will die and how they will recognise dying
- medications, and whether, for example, morphine hastens death.

How long have I (s/he) got?

While it is true that predicting the timing and manner of dying is highly imprecise, as outlined earlier there are well-recognised criteria to identify imminent death from chronic disease.[1] Anecdotally health professionals are often quoted as having been wrong in predicting the end of life: *'they said he only had days to live and ...'*. First, it is important to recognise that when such instances are quoted, reliable information as to what was actually said is often unavailable. Second, particularly in late-stage disease, it is likely that many more such predictions turned out to be broadly accurate. In practice, people do have reasonable expectations of the professionals' willingness to share judgement (not certainty) about prognosis.[5] The need to pass on such judgements to relatives who are away is often a major concern. It may be wise to recognise that the decision to come home is for the relative who is away to balance against other responsibilities and, indeed, pleasures. Relatives caring for the patient can be helped by reassurance that their responsibility is to describe how things are for the patient rather than to make decisions about whether other relatives should return home. Just how important it is for relatives to be present at the precise moment of death can usefully be explored and it is helpful at times to question the significance of what can be an almost imperceptible transition from life to death, without drama or significant 'last words'.

Explaining the appropriate role for drugs

When discontinuing treatments, a positive decision with explanation as to why particular drugs are no longer appropriate is often appreciated. If patients are to continue to feel valued, care must be taken to avoid the unwitting implication that it is just no longer worth continuing with medications – such as hormonal treatments for breast cancer or blood pressure tablets – which may have been previously recommended as lifelong therapy. Equally, a clear judgement should be conveyed about the role of analgesics and sedatives. It is tempting for relatives and others to blame medication for increasing weakness, sleepiness and confusion. A careful assessment of the probabilities, and clear reassurance when drugs are most unlikely to be responsible, is often most helpful. Similarly, reassurance should be given that food and fluid intake in the last days of life is not needed and may indeed be harmful. Specifically it has been shown that biochemically measured dehydration does not correlate with symptoms of thirst.[6]

Honest reassurance

Even when the news is very bad, honest (and therefore powerful) reassurance can usually be given. Surprisingly patients and relatives may fear that dying will be associated with escalating pain, convulsions, bleeding or sheer panic. In a society where many people are unfamiliar with the dying process, sensible ordinary reassurance about these very rare possibilities can be a key role for even the moderately experienced professional.

Ethical issues

Much of good care for the dying is to do with moral judgement rather than scientific competence. The useful and rapid distinction between these two approaches can be made by asking whether the challenge can best be phrased as 'what can we do' (scientific, technical) or 'what should we do' (moral). There is scope in this chapter only to touch on ethical challenges in caring for the dying and to address a few common ethical questions.

'I gave the last injection; did I kill him?'

Fundamental to successful palliative care is a secure understanding of the morally, and legally, sound answer to this question. Whenever the intention is to ease suffering with proportionate use of appropriate medications the answer to the question is *no*. Support from professional colleagues is profoundly important to ensure that limiting patients' suffering remains the prime concern. Whether the doctrine of double effect[7] *(originally a contribution from Catholic morality)* is useful in this area of practice is a matter for debate.[8]

Key tip 9.1

The principle of double effect permits an act, which is foreseen to have both good and bad effects, provided:

- the act itself is good or neutral
- the good effect is the reason for acting
- the good effect is not caused by the bad effect and a proportionate reason exists for causing the bad effect.[9]

Who are we treating?

Where the interests of the patient and the interest of the relatives coincide, the answer is easy. However, the needs of exhausted carers may not always coincide with the patient. While the patient's interests must continue to come first, the autonomous ability or indeed willingness of others to provide for the patient may legitimately limit choice. For instance, previous promises to provide care at home may become untenable. Indeed, despite most people expressing the preference for dying at home, this question is inevitably asked at a time when the patient cannot be certain of all the circumstances and implications of carrying out their wishes. At the moment of greatest reality, many people are ultimately grateful for inpatient care arranged very late in the course of illness.[10] The question of who we are treating arises when, for instance, noisy breathing, or the thought of their loved one dehydrating to death, distresses the family. Most people would wish to spare their relatives unnecessary suffering and in these circumstances it may be justifiable to give treatments such as hyoscine or subcutaneous fluids if it is judged morally neutral for the patient and beneficial for their loved ones.

Is he now too unwell to make or sign a Will?

Professionals will know that willingness to sign as witnesses to the making or signing of a Will implies agreement that the person concerned has the necessary mental capacity. In the last few days of life, this will rarely be the case. The Lord Chief Justice set out the following criteria for testamentary capacity in the case of *Banks v Goodfellow*:

> It is essential ... that a testator shall understand the nature of the Act and its effects; shall understand the property of which he is disposing; shall be able to comprehend and appreciate the claims to which he ought to give effect; and, with a view to the latter object, that no disorder of mind shall poison his affections, pervert his sense of right, or prevent the exercise of his natural faculties – that no insane delusion shall influence his will in disposing of his property and bring about a disposal of it which, if the mind had been sound, would not have been made.

This is still recognised as the most important legal case.[11]

In the light of this, despite understandable efforts to help distressed relatives, an absent or out-of-date Will can rarely be validly put right in the last few days of life.

Conclusion

There are few more satisfying tasks than to assist someone to die comfortably, appropriately and at peace, in a place of their choosing, cared for by those closest to them. While specialist palliative care professionals can and should assist, generalist healthcare professionals can provide satisfactory care at the end of life, given the right support.

Self-assessment exercise 9.1
Time: 30 minutes
1 What are the drug treatments for:
   a Pain?
   b Shortness of breath?
   c Nausea and vomiting?
   d Agitation?
   e Noisy breathing?
2 What concerns may the family have regarding end-of-life issues?
3 Reflect on how you could help the family, living some distance away, to make a decision to visit.
4 What do you understand by the term *'the doctrine of double effect'*?
5 Reflect on your practice in caring for a dying person:
   a Did you feel the experience rewarding, difficult – or both?
   b Consider what made it so.

References

1   Ellershaw JE, Ward C. Care of the dying patient: the last hours or days of life. *BMJ*. 2003; **326**: 30–34.
2   Stevenson J, Abernethy AP, Miller C *et al.* (2004) Managing co-morbidities in patients at the end of life. *BMJ*. 2004; **329**: 909–912.
3   National Council for Hospice and Specialist Palliative Care Services. *Changing Gear: guidelines for managing the last days of life in adults.* December. London: National Council for Hospice and Specialist Palliative Care Services (NCHSPCS); 2001.
4   Boyd KJ, Kelly M. Oral morphine as symptomatic treatment of dyspnoea in patients with advanced cancer. *Palliative Medicine*. 1997; **11**: 277–281.
5   Christakis NA. *Death Foretold: prophecy and prognosis in medical care.* Chicago: University of Chicago Press; 1999.
6   Ellershaw JE, Sutcliffe JM, Saunders CM. Dehydration and the dying patient. *J Pain and Symptom Management*. 1995; **10**(3): 192–197.
7   Gula M (1989) *Reason Informed by Faith; foundations of Catholic morality.* New York: Paulist Press; 1989, pp. 265–282.
8   Gilbert J. Palliative medicine: a new specialty changes an old debate in euthanasia: death, dying and the medical duty. *British Medical Bulletin*. 1996; **52**: 296–397.
9   Gilbert J, Kirkham S. Double effect, double bind or double speak? *Palliative Medicine*. 1999; **13**: 365–366.
10 Boyd KJ. Short terminal admissions to a hospice. *Palliative Medicine*. 1993; **7**: 289–294.
11 British Medical Association and the Law Society. *Assessment of Mental Capacity*, 2nd edition. London: British Medical Association; 2004, p. 33.

To learn more

• Buckman R. *I Don't Know What to Say.* London: Macmillan; 1988.
• Cooper J. Coping with death and bereavement. Basford L, Slevin O, editors. *Theory and Practice of Nursing: an integrated approach to caring practice.* 2nd edition. Cheltenham: Nelson Thornes; 2003, Chapter 35, pp. 664–681.
• Ellershaw J, Wilkinson S. *Care of the Dying: a pathway to excellence.* Oxford: Oxford University Press; 2003.
• Faull C, Carter Y, Woof R. *Handbook of Palliative Care.* Oxford: Blackwell Science; 1998.
• National Council for Hospice and Specialist Palliative Care Services. *Changing Gear: guidelines for managing the last days of life in adults.* December. London: National Council for Hospice and Specialist Palliative Care Services (NCHSPCS); 2001.
• Thomas K. *Caring for the Dying at Home.* Oxford: Radcliffe Medical Press; 2003.

Complementary chapters

See also Stepping into Palliative Care 1: relationships and responses

• Chapter 3: The cancer journey
• Chapter 4: The experience of illness
• Chapter 5: The psychological impact of serious illness
• Chapter 6: Hope and coping strategies
• Chapter 7: The therapeutic relationship
• Chapter 8: Gold Standard Framework: a programme for community palliative care
• Chapter 9: Integrated care pathways

- Chapter 13: Communication: the essence of good practice, management and leadership
- Chapter 14: Ethical dilemmas
- Chapter 15: Transcultural and ethnic issues at the end of life

See also Stepping into Palliative Care 2: care and practice

- Chapter 5: Mouth care
- Chapter 7: Wound care
- Chapter 10: Terminal restlessness
- Chapter 11: Breaking bad news
- Chapter 13: Spirituality and palliative care

Answers to Pre-reading exercise 9.1

- Profoundly weak.
- Usually bedbound.
- Help with care.
- Sleepy.
- Uninterested in food or fluids.
- Difficulty swallowing.

Terminal restlessness

Jo Cooper

Pre-reading exercise 10.1
Time: 30 minutes

Terminal restlessness and delirium presents a challenge for the inter-disciplinary team. Moreover, it presents the family with distress and despair.

Read the *case scenario* then consider the physical, psychological, spiritual and social dimensions. How will Peter's symptoms and illness impact on:

- Peter?
- Mary?
- Paul?
- Jane?

Case scenario 10.1

Peter (56) is married to Mary. They have two children, Paul (20) and Jane (16). Peter was an English teacher who stopped work recently due to treatment for small cell lung cancer. Chemotherapy ceased 6 weeks ago when a scan showed the tumour to be unresponsive.

Mary, a nurse in the chemotherapy unit where Peter received his treatment, stopped work 4 weeks ago when Peter's condition further deteriorated.

Paul is at university some 130 miles from the family home. He is returning home having been told by Mary that his father is deteriorating.

Jane sits her exams in 3 weeks and plans to continue to take her A-levels.

Now Peter is dying. He is agitated, restless, anxious and frightened. He is too weak to stand but continually tries to get out of bed.

Comment
The need to explore the impact of terminal restlessness and the treatment on the family is imperative. The family are often present during the last days or hours of life prior to death. They are closely involved and any decisions relating to care and treatment impacts on them.[1]

Read on – at the end of this chapter return to reflect on your responses.

- *Could you have identified more problems?*
- *What effect might this have on your own emotions?*

What is terminal restlessness?

The terms 'terminal restlessness', 'terminal anguish' and 'delirium' are often used interchangeably. Terminal restlessness overlaps with but is not necessarily identical to delirium.[2]

Terminal restlessness can be defined as the agitation and restlessness that may occur during the last few hours or days of life. Between 68% and 88% of patients may exhibit:[3]

- anxiety
- agitation
- impaired consciousness
- physical irritability
- myoclonus (muscular jerking).[4]

Delirium (aka acute confusional state) may be accompanied by:

- reduced attention
- memory impairment
- disorientation
- hallucinations
- altered perception and misinterpretation
- restlessness
- anxiety
- irritability
- noisy, aggressive behaviour.[5]

Over 80% of advanced cancer patients experience delirium in the final days.[6]

Assessment and goal

Assessment is pivotal to providing safe, effective outcomes in terminal restlessness. It is continuous – not 'one-off'. The *goal* is to:

- *provide* – physical and emotional comfort
- *maintain* – a conscious level that enables family relationships and communication
- *reduce* – the distress of the family.

Terminal restlessness is distressing for the patient and family, and it can be mismanaged through fear of oversedation. Therefore, interdisciplinary, skilled assessment and effective therapeutic intervention maximises symptom relief.

Self-assessment exercise 10.1
Time: 5 minutes

List the causes of terminal restlessness.

Identifying the cause

The causative factors leading to terminal restlessness need to be identified quickly and effectively (*see* Box 10.1). Once recognised, it must be treated.[6] Pain should be excluded as a cause and requires appropriate analgesics.

Box 10.1   Treatable causes of terminal restlessness[4]

- Generalised physical discomfort.
- Bladder or bowel distension.
- Breathlessness.
- Anoxia.
- Nicotine withdrawal — consider nicotine patch or Nicorette nasal spray.
- Alcohol withdrawal — consider diazepam in decreasing doses for 7–10 days.
- Illicit drug withdrawal.
- Infection.
- Drug induced – e.g. opioids, antibiotics, anticonvulsants, digoxin, diuretics, non-steroidal anti-inflammatory drugs (NSAIDs), steroids, hypnotics.
- Dehydration.

When assessing terminal restlessness consider the following factors:

- *opioids* – in 64% of cases[6]
- *cause* – may be multifactorial or not be found.[2,6]
- *discovered cause* – found in less than 50% of patients
- *misdiagnosis* – jeopardises quality of life[7]
- *irreversible cause* – when identified it is often irreversible (e.g. liver failure or cerebral metastases)[2,6]
- *tests* – often inappropriate if time is short or the patient is at home
- *patient communication* – patient may be unable to state the cause of restlessness (e.g. feeling uncomfortable, experiencing pain, feeling afraid).

Precipitating factors of terminal restlessness are listed in Box 10.2.[4]

Box 10.2   Precipitating factors of terminal restlessness[3]

- Cerebral oedema.
- Heart failure.
- Primary brain tumour.
- Cerebral vascular accident (CVA).
- Biochemical imbalance (urea, calcium, sodium, glucose).
- Deteriorating liver and renal function.
- Unresolved psychosocial issues.

As well as assessing and correcting the cause of terminal restlessness or delirium, symptomatic and supportive measures are important for minimising the distress caused to the patient.[6]

The opportunity should be taken to review and discontinue medication where necessary. Drugs frequently cause delirium and agitation. Therefore, it is imperative to check current medication.

Key tip 10.1

It is common to find more than one drug responsible for causing delirium.[6]

Management

Pharmacological therapy and psychological intervention to minimise the distress of the patient and relative(s) are the mainstay of treatment for terminal restlessness. Supportive nursing care includes:

- *environment* – provide a safe environment; if the patient is delirious, there may be a danger to self and others
- *injury* – if appropriate, a mattress placed on the floor, although not ideal, may be a safer option in the acute situation
- *quiet* – encourage a peaceful, quiet environment
- *lighting* – use of soft lighting; fears are often exacerbated at night; low light at night promotes a feeling of safety
- *noise* – reduce levels to aid sleep
- *company* – if appropriate, reassure the patient that someone will stay with them. A member of the family or a familiar friend will help to reduce distress. It is preferable to maintain continuity of care
- *massage* – gentle massage using relaxing essential oils may help to maximise feelings of wellbeing; essential oils, used in a vaporising burner, may provide sensory pleasure and reduce anxiety
- *touch* – can be powerful, alerting the patient to your presence and demonstrating a sense of care
- *explanations* – give simple and clear explanations of what is going to happen and what can be done to help the patient and relatives
- *reassurance* – reassure relatives that terminal restlessness is often part of the process of dying; relatives may feel responsible for the patient's symptoms – a sense that they have 'done something wrong'[4]
- *recuperation* – ensure that relatives have the opportunity for rest and take time to themselves
- *supervision* – increased nursing supervision is essential
- *continuity* – staff continuity is a priority.

Cognitive interventions can apply to the patient and relatives,[7] and can include:

- *communication* – simple and clear
- *acknowledgement* – of the patient's feelings
- *alleviating isolation* – encourage brief family visits

- *fostering a sense of control* – explain interventions
- *balancing hope and reality*.

Pharmacological therapy

Key tip 10.2

Intramuscular (IM) injections are painful for thin, frail patients, and should be avoided. The subcutaneous route is kinder and effective.

Many patients are unable to take oral medication due to their agitated state, fluctuating levels of consciousness or general level of debility. In such instances, the subcutaneous route should be used.

The medication of choice for terminal restlessness without delirium is midazolam (a benzodiazepine).[2] The common dose range of midazolam is 30–60 mg per 24 hours via continuous subcutaneous infusion. Doses of 10 mg per 24 hours can be given with good effect, depending on assessment of condition.

Key tip 10.3

Remember to administer a stat dose of midazolam, 5 mg to 10 mg subcutaneously, prior to setting up the syringe driver. This good practice calms the agitated patient while the syringe driver medication takes effect.

Key tip 10.4

If the patient fails to settle comfortably with midazolam 30 mg/24 hours then introduce haloperidol 5 mg/24 hours *before* increasing midazolam.[8]

Midazolam facts

- Midazolam has a quick-onset action.
- Midazolam is *water-soluble* and it mixes with most of the drugs commonly given by syringe driver.[5]
- In agitated terminal delirium, larger doses are sometimes necessary, especially if anxiety has been a feature, or in the case of a patient who has been using denial as a coping mechanism.[5]
- Tolerance may develop after the patient has shown a good initial response.
- Continual review is pivotal to good management.

Limitations

- *Use a large syringe* – large volumes of the injection are needed when using a high dose.
- *Syringe/pump* – a 20 ml or 30 ml syringe will fit Graseby pumps MS16A and MS26.
- *Change syringe* – if necessary, can be changed 12-hourly instead of 24-hourly.

Diazepam (a benzodiazepine) facts

- Diazepam given as a suppository per rectum (PR) is useful in a crisis.[5] A stat dose of 20 mg, PR and 6- to 8-hourly, may be helpful in such cases.

Self-assessment exercise 10.2
Time: 5 minutes

List the difficulties one might encounter using the rectal route in terminal restlessness.

Limitations

- Rectal administration of diazepam at home may be difficult due to the practical problems of moving and changing position.
- Diazepam can only be used if the patient has given consent (patients' choice).
- There may be problems if the patient is impacted or has diarrhoea. Haemorrhoids, tumour, rectal discharge or pain may also exclude this route.[9]

Levomepromazine (methotrimeprazine – a phenothiazine) facts

- Levomepromazine is often used for agitation.[10]
- A stat dose of 25 mg subcutaneously and 50 to 75 mg/24 hours administered via a syringe driver may be beneficial.[8]
- Depending on the response, titrate the dose.
- Drug action onset – approximately 30 minutes.
- The duration of the dose action is 12–24 hours.[8]
- Levomepromazine can be advantageous because of its antiemetic benefits.[8]
- Levomepromazine is available in 25 mg tablets or as 25 mg in a 1 ml injection.
- If there is a risk of convulsions, midazolam 30 to 60 mg/24 hours can be added.[5]

Haloperidol (a butyrophenone) facts

- Haloperidol is the drug of choice for restlessness *with* delirium.[11,12]
- Oral haloperidol is effective and some patients manage well with this.[2]
- In low doses of 1.5 mg to 3 mg, it is usually effective in targeting:
  - fear
  - agitation
  - paranoia.[2]
- Haloperidol does not induce severe sedation.
- Communication may still be maintained.

- Parenteral doses are approximately twice as potent as the equivalent oral dose.[2]
- Haloperidol can be administered over a 24-hour period via a syringe driver.
- Doses do not generally exceed 20 mg/24 hours.[2]
- The suggested range of haloperidol is:
  - *older patients* – 1.5 to 3 mg stat, and at night (nocte)
  - *younger patients* – 5 mg stat, and at night (nocte)
  - *poor response* – in cases of poor response, give 10 to 30 mg at night (nocte), or in a divided dose.[8]
- It is beneficial to titrate the drug to the behaviour.
- Haloperidol is useful for controlling agitation and improving cognition. *However, if death is likely to occur soon, this may be unachievable.*[2]
- The causes of delirium may be irreversible in the active, dying phase.[2]
- If the delirium cannot be reversed, sometimes it may be necessary to use:
  - *midazolam*
  - *levomepromazine.*

Box 10.3 provides an at-a-glance view of the three regimes.

Box 10.3   Medication for terminal restlessness

Midazolam
Suggested range:[8]
30 mg to 60 mg/24 hours via continuous subcutaneous infusion.
Stat dose:
5 mg to 10 mg subcutaneously will help to calm the agitated patient while syringe-driver medication takes effect.

Levomepromazine
Suggested range:[8,10]
50 mg to 75 mg/24 hours via continuous subcutaneous infusion.
Stat dose:
25 mg subcutaneously.

Haloperidol
Suggested range:[8]
Older patients: 1.5–3 mg stat and at night – orally.
Younger patients: 5 mg stat and at night – orally.
Normal dose: 5 mg/24 hours via continuous subcutaneous infusion.
Usual maximum dose:
5–30 mg/24 hours via continuous subcutaneous infusion.[5]

Psychological interventions

While pharmacological intervention is the mainstay of the control of restlessness, agitation and delirium, psychological support is pivotal in helping to alleviate anxiety and distress.

Key tip 10.5

It is just as important to remember the need for psychological intervention.

Self-assessment exercise 10.3
Time: 15 minutes

- Consider the concept of loss.
- Take time to visualise how you would feel if you lost something or someone precious to you.

Unresolved emotions issues

Unresolved issues in the patient's life can cause restlessness and agitation. Spiritual pain or fear can be resistant to treatment interventions.[4] Spiritual or emotional pain, fear and anger can be withheld and may not be exposed until physical symptoms (e.g. pain, nausea, vomiting) are effectively controlled.

The patient's emotional issues should be explored early, if appropriate, and with the patient's agreement, with the family. As the family's emotional need may be different from the patient's, the opportunity to explore fears and concerns, away from the patient, should be offered. Ensuring a safe environment for such disclosure is essential. It may be necessary to arrange meetings within or outwith the home environment and it should be emphasised that this is possible.

Where appropriate, referral to other professionals and agencies should be made, e.g.:

- counsellor
- clinical psychologist
- family therapist
- minister of religion.

Some individuals do not accept they are dying. Denial can be a means of coping with the end of life. While supporting the patient, and identifying and aiming to reduce distress, there must be respect for the individual's choice. The patient needs to feel safe and have the opportunity to cope in his/her own way. The professional should acknowledge this freedom of choice. However, if emotional distress is not explored, the patient is often unable to control thoughts and unresolved fears that can break through into the confused mind with devastating results.[5]

Supporting the family

Guiding the family, and demonstrating empathy by 'being with' them through this distressing time, is essential. There are no short cuts. Teamwork is vital. Families benefit from a supportive interdisciplinary approach exploring the multifaceted needs of each individual. Families often experience a sense of helplessness and isolation. They may feel 'pushed away' by the patient. It needs to be acknowledged that as the 'professional' it is difficult for us, too, when we come across situations where we feel helpless. Therefore, one can observe and appreciate that, for the family at such times, there is a constant reminder, sustained over weeks or months, that can, if unrecognised, have a detrimental long-term effect on their lives.

Key tip 10.6

See Chapter 7 in *Stepping into Palliative Care 1* to develop your understanding of a relationship that is therapeutic and beneficial.

Sedation should always be discussed with the family. Their views are important and should be explored. The professional should aim to offer clear, straightforward information. Check the relatives' understanding throughout. Make sure the family understand that medication will make the patient feel sleepy, rendering verbal communication difficult. Listen to what is said, and what is not said. Give time and opportunity for each family member to express individual concerns and the issues that are important to them.

A study of relatives of patients who experienced terminal restlessness identified five themes that described the impact on them:

- the multidimensionality of suffering
- the need for communication
- the feelings of ambivalence
- the need for information
- the need for sensitivity and respect.[1]

Family time

Reassure the family that time set aside for them is important and that it is acceptable to take that time. Taking care of oneself is pivotal in enabling the care of the patient. Families often feel guilty about spending time on themselves. There is the feeling that 'personal time' can take them away from what they perceive they should be doing (i.e. looking after the patient).

Using supportive complementary therapies, and attending a support group, may be appropriate. Agencies within the family's local community may provide 'home carers' who can stay with the patient while the family member shops, visits the hairdressers or attends to their own healthcare needs.

Aiming to be honest

Colluding with the frightened, dying patient that they will get better and 'everything will be all right' is not helpful. It is easy for the family and the professional to collude with the patient when they are unsure about what to say or do. Colluding may serve to undervalue their feelings, and blocks *any* useful communication, thus making 'letting go' difficult.

Listen carefully to the patient's and family's fears, concerns and questions. Watch for non-verbal communication, and be calm and genuine. Be yourself. Show that you understand and that you are there – be with them. This enhances the therapeutic relationship. Clever words and phrases are inappropriate and unnecessary. The unspoken, the silence and the 'being with' can all offer comfort to the dying person.

Sometimes the patient needs to be 'given permission' to die by the family. People often wish to hold on to what they know and love. It can be a struggle for both parties to let go. It is sometimes sufficient for the family to tell the patient that it is all right for them to die.[13]

Dying may give rise to many repressed emotions: sadness, numbness, guilt, and jealousy of those who are well.[14] It is often helpful to the family for them to understand that being open and honest with the patient can open up channels of communication. This may be helped by facilitation by an appropriate professional. Often merely asking the patient 'how' they, the family, can help may be useful. The patient is sometimes able to give the family help and guidance in meeting their needs.

Conclusion

Terminal restlessness and agitation, with or without delirium, is a frightening experience. It represents a challenge. Ongoing assessment and evaluation is central to achieving effective outcomes. Constant monitoring, using a team approach, is needed to enable rapid, effective and therapeutic responses to any change.

Preparing the family for the possible occurrence of restlessness and agitation may be a possibility. Reassurance that, in most cases, something can be done will help to reduce some of the inevitable anxieties, and is essential. Being prepared for possible events leading up to the patient's death may help the patient and family to cope better. If the family have some awareness and understanding that such events are sometimes part of dying, and not due to negligence in the care given to the patient, this may make it easier to talk the issue through with other relatives and help to minimise the extreme distress and difficulties that can occur.

Dying is not always peaceful. Although it should always be the aim of the professional, realistically it is not always possible. It is important that the professional takes care of his/her own needs, and those of colleagues with whom we work.

Key tip 10.7

Clinical supervision is a helpful way to explore one's own feelings within the context of a challenging situation.

The following are essential for effective therapeutic intervention.

- *Be realistic* – about what can be achieved.
- *Whole picture* – consider the whole picture encapsulating physical, psychological, spiritual and social dimensions.

- *Professional update* – continually update knowledge with research and evidence-based practice.
- *Maximum skills* – maximise the use of intuitive and factual skills and knowledge.
- *Limitations* – it is acceptable to acknowledge our own limitations.

Conceptualising and embracing the above enables the professional to provide a high quality standard of care and maximises support for the patient and family. Pharmacological *and* non-pharmacological therapies play an important role in the management of terminal restlessness in palliative care.

Patients and family are:

- real people
- facing real problems and traumatic situations
- often with limited resources of their own.

As professionals, we must respect the individual. Time must be given to:

- *listen* – to what is said
- *observe* – what is not said
- *provide* – the highest standard of care and expertise that is available.

It is imperative that we listen to people as individuals, for they are the true experts.

Self-assessment exercise 10.4
Time: 20 minutes

1 How would you define terminal restlessness?
2 List three possible treatable causes of terminal restlessness.
3 What practical support can be given to the patient?
4 What is the drug of choice for terminal restlessness without delirium?
5 What is the drug of choice for terminal restlessness with delirium?
6 List three emotions that may be repressed by the dying person.

Now list what support you can give to the family and/or carer during this difficult time.
(*See* answers on page 169.)

References

1 Brajtman S. The impact on the family of terminal restlessness and its management. *Palliative Medicine.* 2003; **17**: 454–460.
2 Breitbart W, Chochinovov HM, Passik S. Psychiatric aspects of palliative care. In: Doyle D, Hanks GWC, MacDonald N, editors. *Oxford Textbook of Palliative Medicine,* 2nd edition. Oxford: Oxford University Press; 1998.
3 Lawlor PG, Gagnon B, Mancini IL *et al.* Occurrence, causes and outcomes of delirium in patients with advanced cancer. *Arch Int Med.* 2000; **160**: 786–794.
4 March PA. Hospice techniques: terminal restlessness. *Am J Hospice Palliative Care.* 1998; **Jan/Feb**: 51–53.
5 Twycross R. *Symptom Management in Advanced Cancer,* 3rd edition. Oxford: Radcliffe Medical Press; 2001.
6 Centeno C, Sanz A, Bruera E. Delirium in advanced cancer patients. *Palliative Medicine.* 2004; **18**: 184–194.

7   Brown S, Degner LF. Delirium in the terminally ill cancer patient: aetiology, symptoms and management. *Int J of Palliative Nursing*. 2001; **7**(6): 266–272.

8   Twycross R, Wilcock A, Charlesworth S *et al*. *PCF2 Palliative Care Formulary*, 2nd edition. Oxford: Radcliffe Medical Press; 2002.

9   De Sousa E, Jepson BA. Midazolam in terminal care. *The Lancet*. 1988; **i**: 67–68.

10   Oliver DJ. The use of methotrimeprazine in terminal care. *Br J Clin Practice*. 1995; **39**: 339–340.

11   Mazzocato C, Stiefel F, Buclin T *et al*. Psychopharmacology in supportive care of cancer: a review for the clinician. *Neuroleptics Support Care Cancer*. 2000; **8**: 89–97.

12   Breitbart W, Strout D. Delirium in the terminally ill. *Clinics Ger. Med*. 2000; **16**(2): 357–372.

13   Callahan C, Kelly P. *Final Gifts*. New York: Poseidon Press; 1992.

14   Rinpoche S. *The Tibetan Book of Living and Dying*. London: Ryder; 1998.

To learn more

- Callahan C, Kelly P. *Final Gifts*. New York: Poseidon Press; 1992.
- Cooper J. Coping with death and bereavement. In: Basford L, Slevin O, editors. *Theory and Practice of Nursing: an integrated approach to caring practice*. Cheltenham: Nelson Thornes; 2003, Chapter 35.
- Doyle D, Hanks GW, MacDonald N. *Oxford Textbook of Palliative Medicine*. Oxford: Oxford University Press; 1998.
- McMahon R, Pearson A. *Nursing As Therapy*, 2nd edition. London: Chapman and Hall; 1998.
- Rinpoche S. *The Tibetan Book of Living And Dying*. London: Rider; 1998.
- Twycross R. *Symptom Management in Advanced Cancer*. 3rd edition. Oxford: Radcliffe Medical Press; 2001.
- Twycross R, Wilcock A, Charlesworth S *et al*. *PCF2 Palliative Care Formulary*. 2nd edition. Oxford; Radcliffe Medical Press; 2002.

Complementary chapters

See also Stepping into Palliative Care 1: relationships and responses

- Chapter 6: Hope and coping strategies
- Chapter 7: The therapeutic relationship
- Chapter 11: The value of teamwork
- Chapter 15: Transcultural and ethnic issues at the end of life

See also Stepping into Palliative Care 2: care and practice

- Chapter 2: Introduction to pain management
- Chapter 4: Continuous subcutaneous infusion
- Chapter 13: Spirituality and palliative care

Answers to Self-assessment exercise 10.4

1 The agitation and restlessness that may occur in the last few hours or days of life.

2

- Physical discomfort.
- Bladder or bowel distension.
- Breathlessness.
- Anoxia.
- Nicotine withdrawal.
- Alcohol withdrawal.
- Illicit drug withdrawal.
- Infection.
- Other drugs.
- Dehydration.

3

- Provision of a safe environment.
- A mattress on the floor.
- A peaceful, quiet environment.
- Use of soft lighting, with low lights at night.
- Continuity of carers and a familiar friend or family member to stay with the patient.
- Gentle massage with relaxing oils.
- Appropriate use of touch.
- Providing information and an explanation to the family.

4 Midazolam.
5 Haloperidol.
6 Sadness, numbness, guilt, jealousy (of those who are well).

Now that you have read this chapter, you may be able to think of other approaches you could use. The important thing to remember is to be you. Be genuine in your responses.

Chapter 11

Breaking bad news

Mezzi Franklin

It is impossible to cure all patients; that would be an achievement surpassing in difficulty even the forecasting of future developments. (Hippocrates, 330 BC)[1]

Pre-reading exercise 11.1
Time: 15 minutes

When breaking bad news, or supporting an individual who has received bad news, the first step is to be aware of our own feelings. If we cannot understand ourselves in this situation, we are unlikely to understand the feelings and needs of the patient and family we speak to.

Before reading this chapter:

- Think about the feelings that you may experience when you discover that you have lost something. Perhaps it is your car keys and you are about to go to an important meeting, or you are at the checkout in a supermarket and you have lost your debit card.
- Write down your feelings. Compare with those identified in this chapter.

Introduction

This chapter is divided in to three parts:

- *preparation* – for breaking bad news
- *strategies* – for breaking bad news
- *resources* – that may be useful in dealing with the effects of bad news.

Preparation for breaking bad news

Understanding why breaking bad news is so difficult

Breaking bad news is distressing, painful and difficult for professionals. This may be because we enter into the caring professions to try and make things better for people.[2] Telling an individual they have cancer or a life-limiting illness works against this. As professionals, we are left in the difficult position of trying to say something helpful in a situation that, at best, offers uncertain hope of cure.

In the healthcare setting, it is still considered good practice not to show emotion.[3] This can result in a juxtaposition of breaking bad news in a cold and clinical way to someone who is overcome with emotion. We may be fearful of '*letting ourselves go*' by showing how we really feel. Balancing this against the emotion we know we are about to evoke can result in a situation where we break bad news quickly to protect ourselves from the emotional response of the patient.

No person with cancer can be promised that they are cured or that the cancer will never return. That is a painful realisation for patient, family and professional. This knowledge can result in the fear of '*being blamed*' by the patient for the illness.[4] It may feel kind to promise that the cancer has been treated, and will never return. However, if we are to gain the patient and family's trust, we have to be honest and trustworthy.[5] It is often the nurse that the patient and family turn to and ask '*Can you explain what the doctor said?*' because they trust him/her.

Looking after ourselves

As professionals, we tend to view the importance of our self-care as a luxury that should take a back seat when caring for the patient and family. However, if we do not look after ourselves, we may not be able to care for the patient and family, because of exhaustion. When approaching an accident, the first thing professionals are taught is to ask: 'Is it safe to approach?' In the same way, when considering breaking bad news, and dealing with the effects of bad news, we need to carry out a personal assessment. In this way, we can:

- *Be aware* – of how we are feeling.
- *Assess* – if we are in the right frame of mind to carry out the task. Is there anything that will help focus our attention and promote an objective, supportive approach? If not, are we the right person for the task?
- *Ask* – are we the right person to provide the information? While being emotionally prepared for the task we may still not be the right person. It is important to acknowledge this and hand over to another colleague if s/he has a greater understanding of the situation.
- *Check* – are we prepared? Do we have all the information concerning the case? Are we familiar with the patient's story? If not, gather all the information before approaching the patient.
- *Remember* – the patient's story, however sad, belongs to them, not us. We can work alongside the patients and family and support them to the best of our ability. However, we do not *own* the story.

By practising the above, we avoid being engulfed in the individual's personal sorrow, and thus rendering ourselves less able to support empathically and constructively.

How we feel

To be given a life-limiting diagnosis is devastating. The individual experiences a barrage of conflicting emotions that can lead to emotional turmoil. If we understand these feelings, we are better equipped to support the patient and family. When we lose something precious or vital to us, we may experience the following emotions:

- shock
- frustration

- anger
- despair
- blaming others
- tears
- gradual acceptance
- forming another way forward.

Self-assessment exercise 11.1
Time: 5 minutes

Compare your list from Pre-reading exercise 11.1 to this one. Are there any similarities?

These emotions have been described as stages of bereavement, and are some of the feelings that patient and family may experience when they have received bad news. We cannot imagine what the person in this position is feeling. It is not possible to say, '*I understand exactly how you are feeling.*' Anyone attempting this will experience a negative response from the individual s/he is trying to help. We cannot know *how* a person is feeling because *we are not that individual*. However, understanding some of the emotion being experienced will enable us to empathise with the patient and family. These are not alien feelings; we encounter them in our everyday life.

Strategies in breaking bad news and dealing with the effects of bad news

There are two parts to breaking bad news:

- the actual breaking of the bad news
- dealing with the effects of the bad news.

It is usually the general practitioner, or the hospital senior clinician, who informs the patient of the diagnosis. However, there are times when another professional will break the news. It may be that the patient feels most comfortable with this person and has chosen to ask them to explain the diagnosis. These situations can happen unexpectedly, and catch the professional unawares. In this situation, communication with the wider team is essential, while acknowledging that the patient may want us to discuss the diagnosis because they feel comfortable with us.

The theory of breaking bad news and the practicalities achieving these goals are often difficult to meet. However, if we have

- the knowledge and skills that are required to perform this task
- guidelines to work from

we can undertake this sensitively and supportively. Patients are likely to live with the illness in a positive way, and emotionally recover quickly, when supported at the time of breaking bad news.[6] However, there is evidence that we are still getting it wrong, particularly in clarity of language.[7] Communication skills training is essential in order to improve the patient's experience of receiving information about their illness.[8]

Hospitals holding a cancer status should provide guidelines for healthcare professionals who are communicating bad news. This is now a mandatory requirement.[9] Training that meets the needs of each specific area regarding patient contact is crucial. This ensures good communication flows at all points of access to healthcare experienced by the patient.[10]

Numerous guidelines and models of breaking bad news exist. The guidelines in this chapter follow a ten-step approach to breaking bad news. This is intended to be an aide-mémoire and covers the basic principles required in breaking bad news (*see* Box 11.1).

Box 11.1   Basic principles in breaking bad news

1   *Introductions* – establish that the patient and any person with them knows your name and your role. Sit down, and ensure that everyone present is sitting at the same level. Maintain eye contact. Be aware of body language.

2   *Revisit the patient's history* – 'Mr Smith, you will remember that you have been experiencing these symptoms ...'

3   *The warning shot* – 'We now have the results of the biopsy, and I can explain to you what we have found.'

4   *Check understanding* – has the patient followed what you are saying? Has the 'warning shot' been acknowledged?

5   *Second warning shot* – advise the patient that the situation is serious. 'I am afraid that the results have shown that there is something serious ...'

6   *Silence* – give the patient and family time to acknowledge the 'warning shot'. Check that they are ready for you to continue.

7   *Explain* – the diagnosis and possible treatment. Use language that is accessible to the patient. Avoid jargon. Use the word 'cancer' if this is the diagnosis.

8   *Give further information* – but do not give more information than the patient can absorb.

9   *Support* – offer further support to the patient and family. If in outpatients, do they want input from the specialist nurse, if they are not present? Follow up/ support at home. Would they like input from the clinical nurse specialist in palliative care?

10   *Time out* – would the patient and family like some quiet time on their own?

Step approach to breaking bad news

There are five pivotal preparatory steps to enable breaking bad news:

- *Preparation* – is all the appropriate information available?
- *Support* – does the patient wish to have a family member present?

- *Privacy* – have you identified a quiet, private area where you can talk to the patient and family?
- *Interruptions* – have you turned off your bleep, diverted the phone? Have you communicated with colleagues that you do not wish to be disturbed?
- *Awareness* – do the patient and family know that you are going to explain the diagnosis?

Preparation

It can be easy to rush into situations without the relevant information. This usually happens if we are caught unawares and not expecting that particular question at that time. Remember, the patient may have waited for a number of days for investigation results and will want access to all the information relating to the diagnosis. However, it is acceptable to explain that more time is needed to gather all the information in order to help them understand.

Support

In an ideal world, we should know if the patient wants a family member with them when given information about their condition before we are at the stage of breaking bad news. Unfortunately, it is often not until this situation is reached that we ask about support. This is likely to act as a 'warning shot' for the patient as they may wonder why they might need to have a relative with them. It is important to identify any support structure that the patient may want at the outset. Explain that this is routine, and every patient is asked this question.

Privacy

It may be difficult to find a quiet and comfortable area to break bad news, but it is *essential* to try. While the GP's surgery may be more user-friendly, it is often in the hospital setting that the bad news is broken. If a patient is on a ward, and too ill to move, then the best that can be offered is to pull the curtains around the bed. While this non-verbal action acknowledges that we respect the patients' privacy, it should be remembered that curtains are not walls or doors.

Interruptions

In our society, technological communication can override the physical presence. Anyone who has been silenced by the telephone interrupting conversation and taking priority will know how frustrating it is. Therefore, before commencing contact with the patient and family:

- *check* – bleeps and telephones are diverted
- *ask* – colleagues not to disturb you.

This enables the patient and family to receive direct attention.

Sometimes, even when we have made all the checks, we are still interrupted by a person walking in who does not think the large 'DO NOT DISTURB' sign applies to them! This reinforces that life is always spiralling forwards and we need to reinforce that every individual, no matter what is wrong with them, is important.

Awareness

The final part of the preparation is to ensure that the patient and family know that we are going to talk with them at this time about the findings of the investigations and diagnosis.

The process of breaking bad news

The five points below focus on the breaking of bad news.

Body language

Ninety-four per cent of direct communication is non-verbal.[11] It is important to remember that the patient and family pick up information from body language.[12] It is essential to maintain eye contact with the patient and family when giving distressing information. The non-verbal message of direct eye contact is saying: '*I am not afraid to stay with you. I will support you. I am here.*'

When talking with people, conversation flows easily if attention is paid to body language. To encourage ease of dialogue:

- sit at the same level
- maintain an open body language; try not to cross arms or legs.

You may find yourself mirroring the patient's body language. This is a signal that effective communication is happening.

By transferring these everyday skills to breaking bad news, conversation with the patient and family may be easier.

Self-assessment exercise 11.2
Time: 15 minutes

We all have an (invisible) space around us. Depending on the person approaching, the amount of space we require can be small or large, e.g. a partner would be able to sit very close without invading our personal space. If a stranger enters the space as close our partner, we feel uncomfortable and move/step back to increase the space.

The next time you are out in mixed company, try to be aware of your space.

- Who do you let close?
- Who do you keep out?
- What actions do you take to increase the space if someone gets too close?

Space

Individuals have different feelings regarding how much personal space they need to feel safe:

- *seating* – allow the patient and family to choose their own seat
- *adjustments* – invite the patient and family to move seating so they are comfortable.

Preparing to break bad news

The preparation should include repeating the history of what has been happening to the patient. This prepares them for the news and ensures that we are aware of their understanding of the situation so far. It can be a preliminary warning shot. Some patients prefer directness and accelerate the conversation to the point where bad news is broken. They may even feel irritated with you for taking so long to get to the point. While this can be frustrating for the patient, it is easier and less emotionally damaging to speed up breaking bad news than it is to slow it down. It is essential that we gauge and progress the information at the pace set by the patients. The amount of information the patient wants may change during the process of breaking bad news. Careful assessment of verbal and non-verbal messages from the patient and family can help us support individual needs

Breaking the news

Simple accessible language is essential. Use the word *'cancer'* if this is the diagnosis. It is not kinder to say *'lump'*, *'growth'* or *'tumour'*. It may feel easier to use these words, but the patient will not necessarily relate these to cancer. In the worst scenario, the patient will think that the news is good, and that the *'lump'* is so insignificant that it does not even require surgery or it can be *'cut out'* and all will be well.

It is tempting to impart as much information as possible. We have discharged our duty, and can go away feeling we have done good work. When given bad news, it is unlikely that the patient will remember everything. More probable is that the patient will latch onto key words and link these to a different context. Therefore, by offering too much information we risk confusing the patient. Except, how much is too much? Every person is different. Every person responds to bad news differently. The best way forward is to:

- *ask* – the patient and be led by what they want
- *assess* – the level of understanding
- *identify* – information to meet the needs of the patient.

Some people will want:

- *booklets* – to take away and absorb
- *websites* – the CancerBACUP website is informative, reliable and accessible in terms of language (www.cancerbacup.org.uk)
- *addresses* – for support and information
- *to ask questions* – related directly or indirectly to the diagnosis

- *to revisit* – the patient may ask for specific points to be repeated or repeatedly check the diagnosis.

Time out

Some people will be shocked by the bad news and may value time alone with their family to try and make some sense of what has been said.

Pivotal areas for action after breaking bad news include:

- *time* – give the time that is needed by the patient and family to gain control before they leave the ward or department
- *reflection* – give the opportunity to discuss any points or questions the patient or family may have
- *support* – give information about access to clinical nurse specialists, hospice, hospital or community care and resources
- *clarify* – give information on what will happen next and who will be involved
- *organise* – support services, appointments and support material
- *general practitioner* – contact the GP, and update on all the agreed outcomes and actions.

The GP is often left out at this time. While the consultant will write, a telephone call to the family doctor provides extra support to the patient and promotes good communication between hospital and community. If community nurses and clinical nurse specialists in palliative care are already involved, it is essential to communicate with them to ensure a continuum of effective care and support.

Resources for dealing with the effects of bad news

We have explored the feelings that individuals may have when given bad news. This is where knowledge of these may be useful. Often the GP or senior hospital doctor breaks bad news, and other professionals later deal with the effects of the bad news. In these circumstances, having the other professional present when bad news is broken is beneficial. The other professional will recognise when the patient has taken information out of context. When supporting the patient or family at this time, the following strategies may be helpful:

- *Understanding* – does the patient and family fully understand everything that has been said?
- *Checking* – does the patient and family want you to go over anything they have been told?
- *Filling in the gaps* – is there anything else that the patient and family want to ask?
- *Silence* – use it effectively.

Understanding

The professional is a useful resource for the patient and family. The initial consultation can leave them feeling shocked. Now that the patient and family have had time to reflect, they are trying to deal with the effects of the bad news. This is when good communication is crucial. What is explained to the patient and family now will be remembered. We are reinforcing what they have been told. Checking under-standing of what has been said provides further opening for the patient and family to ask more. If they feel that they have understood everything, we can still offer the opportunity to talk by checking that they have all the information they want at this time. If the patient or family want to close the meeting and wish us to leave, it is important to recognise and accept that they have had enough. However, leave contact numbers in case they change their mind. This may be the hospital specialist nurse, the Macmillan clinical nurse specialist or community professional.

Silence

When a patient or family is silent, it is tempting to fill the silence with dialogue. However, silence is crucial. They may be thinking about what they have been told, and what this means to them. If the professional intrudes on this silence, the train of thought may be broken at a significant time for them. Wait for them to speak again. Avoid breaking or rushing silence.

Self-assessment exercise 11.3
Time: 5 minutes

Sit in silence with a friend for 2 minutes. Those 2 minutes will feel much longer.

   This gives us an idea of how long silence can feel when, in reality, it is only a minute in time.

Conclusion

Breaking bad news is a difficult part of the professional's role. It presents a challenge, with benefits, risks and opportunities for self-reflection. Sharing the difficulties we experience, within the context of clinical supervision, can reduce concerns around this type of communication.

   If we sit alongside the patient and family and provide support, we are likely to help unravel misunderstanding and promote a way forward for the patient and family that is clear.

Self-assessment exercise 11.4
Time: 20 minutes

Read the following scenario. Using the step-by-step approach, think:

• How would you break bad news to this patient?
• How would you provide support when dealing with the effects of the bad news?

Case scenario 11.1

Mrs Smith (78). She lives alone and has a history of arthritis, which is very debilitating. She is widowed, but has a very supportive daughter, who lives locally. She has been having investigations for a persistent cough and short-ness of breath. Mrs Smith collapsed at home and was admitted to hospital with a severe chest infection. The investigations identified that she has non-small cell lung cancer. The cancer is advanced and surgery is not possible. Other treatment options are to be discussed with the oncologist. Mrs Smith wants to know the outcome of the tests; she was due to go to outpatients this week but her hospital admission has prevented this happening. Mrs Smith states that she feels comfortable with you, and would like you to tell her all the information that you have regarding her investigations.

References

1 Lloyd GER, editor. *Hippocratic Writings*, 2nd edition. London: Penguin Classics; 1992.
2 Kearney M. *Mortally Wounded*. Dublin: Marino Books; 1996.
3 Maguire GP. Breaking bad news: explaining cancer diagnosis and prognosis. *MJA*. 1999; **171**: 288–289.
4 Buckman R. *How to Break Bad News*. 2nd edition. London: Pan Books; 1994.
5 Nursing and Midwifery Council. *Code of Professional Conduct*. London: Nursing and Midwifery Council; 2004.
6 Buckman R. Communications and emotions. *BMJ*. 8 September 2002; **325**: 7366.
7 Cancer Research UK. *Doctors Using Confusing Language In Cancer Consultations*. London: Cancer Research; 2003.
8 Department of Health. *Manual for Cancer Services*. London: Department of Health Publications; 2004. http://www.dh.gov.uk/PublicationsAndStatistics/Publications/PublicationsPolicyAnd Guidance/PublicationsPolicyAndGuidanceArticle/fs/en?CONTENT_ID=4090081&chk=hq28gu.
9 National Institute for Health and Clinical Excellence (NICE). *Improving Supportive and Palliative Care for People with Cancer: guidance on cancer services – the manual*. London: National Institute for Health and Clinical Excellence (NICE); March 2004. www.nice.org.uk/page.aspx?o=home.
10 Department of Health. *The Knowledge and Skills Framework and the Development Review Process*. London: Department of Health Publications; October 2004.
11 Givens DB. *The Nonverbal Dictionary of Gestures, Signs and Body Language Cues*. Spokane, Washington: Center for Nonverbal Studies Press; 2005.
12 Webb C, Wood M. Communication and assessment. In: Dougherty L, Lister S. *The Royal Marsden Hospital Manual of Clinical Nursing Procedures*, 6th edition. London: Blackwell; 2005, Chapter II, pp. 16–42.

To learn more

• Buckman R. *How to Break Bad News*. London: Pan Books; 1994.
• The A-M. *Palliative Care and Communication: the experiences in the clinic*. Buckingham: Open University Press; 2002.
• Breaking Bad News Website. www.breakingbadnews.co.uk.

Complementary chapters

See also Stepping into Palliative Care 1: relationships and responses

- Chapter 2: What is palliative care?
- Chapter 3: The cancer journey
- Chapter 4: The experience of illness
- Chapter 5: The psychological impact of serious illness
- Chapter 6: Hope and coping strategies
- Chapter 7: The therapeutic relationship
- Chapter 12: Stress issues in palliative care
- Chapter 13: Communication: the essence of good practice, management and leadership
- Chapter 15: Transcultural and ethnic issues at the end of life

See also Stepping into Palliative Care 2: care and practice

- Chapter 1: Assessment in palliative care
- Chapter 12: Hearing the pain of the carer
- Chapter 13: Spirituality and palliative care

Hearing the pain of the carer

Mandy Redgrove and Audrey Smyth

Case scenario 12.1

Tom is facing a life-threatening illness. He has cancer, and although his family, friends and colleagues do not, they too are facing this disease. All of them – Tom's child, grandchild, partner and friends – are confronted with death, fear and loss, and for Tom and everyone in his world, life has changed.

Introduction

You are invited to explore how, in the work you do, you might help the people who relate in one way or another to a person like Tom. The aim is to share:

- knowledge and experience gained from listening to many people who are close to someone with a life-threatening disease
- how a person in this position might feel
- what they might need
- what is necessary for you to go at least some way towards meeting that need.

What follows is based on the experiences of the authors as therapists in health and social work settings.

Who is *the carer?*

The term 'carer' may not always be acceptable because it tends to be associated with a patient's physical care. Therefore, it is important to be aware of Tom as more than a physical being. Only then does the notion of caring broaden. The carer is someone who, through a relationship with Tom, can recognise his value as a human being and so restore his spirit and sense of self-worth. In this chapter, the carer is Mary. However, this could describe anyone, of either sex or any relationship, that is significant to Tom, including young adults and children.

Who is suffering?

Usually, Mary will say, *'What have I got to complain about? After all, it's Tom who is ill and facing his death … he must come first.'* Tom may well return home from having treatment at the hospital and say, '*You know, I ought to be thankful. A person I met in the hospital was having a much worse time than me.*'

This tendency to see pain and suffering relatively may be a way of trying to minimise it in order to make it a little more bearable. Although it is always possible to find another human being who can be perceived as being worse off, in the end, these comparisons provide no lasting comfort.

When working with carers, it is important not to collude with their trivialisation of the pain and suffering they inevitably experience. It is much healthier for the carer to have room and encouragement to express what is really going on inside – the fears, frustration and helplessness.

So in answer to the question '*Who is suffering?*' it could be suggested that it is Tom and all those around him. Suffering is suffering. There is no pecking order, and everyone's needs count. This approach fosters the idea that Tom and Mary can come together in an equal, open and reciprocal relationship, rather than Mary martyring herself and making it impossible for Tom to give anything to her. That situation would lead to Tom feeling isolated, redundant and a burden, and Mary feeling trapped and unable to acknowledge her own feelings and needs.

What might the carer feel?

It is very likely that Mary will feel a need to be strong and positive for Tom. She will feel responsible for keeping him and his hope alive. It is also likely that she does not dare to contemplate the possibility that he might die. Even if she does acknowledge this, the prospect may be frightening.

Mary could be facing a spiritual crisis of her own. It is possible that she has not faced her own mortality and that she finds it disturbing. In turn, she will avoid Tom's need to address his death, suffering and what his life has meant. This drives a wedge of unease and discomfort between them and both are left floundering alone in spiritual distress.

Mary feels lost and isolated. Due to Tom's protection of her, and her own protection of him, communication in any meaningful sense ceases. She feels that the relationship with Tom has been lost. Indeed, if the relationship has been a physically intimate one, this emotional distance may well be mirrored in a lack of physical and sexual contact. The sexual relationship may be further complicated if the disease has affected Tom's physical appearance, his body image and his mobility. Mary may feel emotionally and physically distant at a time when she and Tom need each other most.

In this sea of uncertainty and isolation, it is understandable that Mary may become self-doubting and unsure about how to get it right for Tom. People speak of a feeling of 'treading on eggshells', of being fearful of speaking about anything important – like the diagnosis, the future, or what to tell the children. The fear is that to speak of such things might make everything worse.

The stress and tension that results from bottling up these feelings often give rise to anger and an acute sense of helplessness. Many people have described how they have expressed this frustration by being short-tempered and, subsequently, have felt guilty, particularly when their anger has been directed at their dying relative.

Often Mary will feel a tremendous responsibility for Tom's physical wellbeing and treatment. There are countless decisions to be made about:

- when and where to seek medical attention
- how to obtain information
- which treatment option to pursue
- what Tom should eat.

Trying to make such decisions can place a tremendous strain on the relationship.

These responsibilities are in addition to any physical nursing that may be required. Exhaustion is common and is often followed by a feeling of failure and inability to cope. What at first seems like the obvious solution – handing over to someone else – is fraught with difficulty. Mary, understandably, may not want to relinquish her role to someone who will not be able to care for Tom in the way that she does. There is no respite if Mary is consumed with anxiety and sadness whenever she is away from Tom. In addition, it is common for patients like Tom to want only the person they know intimately to care for them. It may be an important opportunity for the expression of physical tenderness, particularly where the situation has had a negative impact on their sexual relationship.

Young adults and children also feel many of the feelings experienced by adult carers. Adults who, by attempting to protect them, often exclude them from the reality of an illness, can make their situation worse. Such exclusion increases anxiety and helplessness. This chapter is concerned with how you can support an adult carer, but the concept is just as relevant to the young adult and child. However, it will be necessary for you to feel comfortable providing creative activities through which young children can communicate their feelings and concerns.

What might the carer need?

Mary is facing a painful experience. Tom, whom she loves, is ill with a life-threatening disease. What does she need? And what might she do to cope with her situation? When something triggers her feeling of fear and loneliness, she will probably try to avoid this pain by self-distraction and pulling away from what she feels. She may do this by concentrating on the need to appear strong for Tom, by keeping busy, or by watching television. Most of us can identify the coping strategies we use ourselves, and sometimes they are necessary and useful for getting through the practicalities of daily life.

This scenario can be seen more clearly in Figure 12.1. The arrows represent Mary repeatedly touching the painful experience and then pulling away from it. She avoids feelings, sometimes for practical reasons, but more often because she fears that if she starts crying she will never stop and that she might crack up and be of no use to anyone. In Figure 12.1, there is no sense of movement, except round in circles. Indeed, there is a sense of holding on *to* the pain, almost of closing around it in fear.

In Figure 12.2, rather than Mary recoiling from her experience, she allows herself to feel it completely. There is a sense of movement through these feelings, and of release and relief. For this to happen, Mary needs the support of a relationship with someone who is unafraid of her negative feelings, who is able to hold her through them, and who is confident of the healing power of their expression. Such a relationship provides Mary with the encouragement, permission and safety to let go of what she feels.*

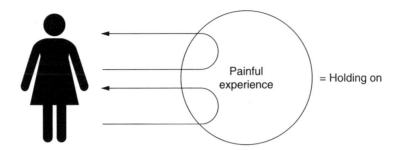

Figure 12.1   Coping by self-distraction and avoiding feelings.

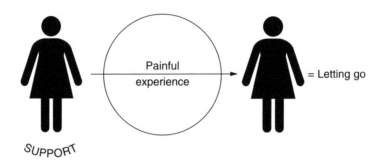

Figure 12.2   Coping by expression of *negative* feelings.

The establishment of this accepting, supporting relationship is absolutely fundamental to the work you do to accompany someone in Mary's position through this turbulent time.

Many issues will come up for her. Examples might include:

- Why is this happening to us?
- What do I believe in?
- What is death?
- Should I give up work?
- How will we manage financially?
- What should we tell the children?
- How can I talk to Tom about dying?
- What about making a will and arranging a funeral?
- How can I support Tom when he goes to see the consultant?
- What treatments should Tom opt for?
- What if Tom loses hope and feels despair?
- What if Tom is in pain?

---

* This model was shared with us by Bill Sandhu, a dear friend who taught us most of what we know about working alongside people.

By listening and helping Mary explore these issues, you provide her with an opportunity to see the whole situation, including her part in it, more clearly. She will feel steadier and less agitated. Because of her work with you, she is more likely to enjoy an open and honest relationship with Tom where difficulties and feelings are shared and unfinished business is dealt with. Helping Mary to use this limited time as effectively as possible means that she and Tom will experience a richer relationship. It will also prevent her from having to live with regrets after Tom has died. In essence, what Mary really needs is for you to enter her world and be alongside her.

Mary will need knowledge of organisations that can provide her with information, services and practical resources. There are organisations that operate nationally. It is advisable to find out about any local services (e.g. hospice) which could offer support, equipment, respite and therapies.

What does it take for you, the professional, to support the carer?

To answer this question, you will probably consider what you could do to support the carer. Yet, if you look at your own experience of being well supported, it is likely to have been as much to do with *how* that person behaved towards you as to anything they may have done practically.

Self-assessment exercise 12.1
Time: 20 minutes

- Reflect on what it means to be in a state where you are open to another human being.
- Write down some adjectives to describe this state.

So, what does it take to support Mary? You, the professional, need to be open hearted. In this place, your heart is open to the present moment, shared with the other. Your mind has no goal; there is no pressure within you to achieve anything. There is a heightened sensitivity and awareness of the human connection between you. From a still, unhurried place within you, responses naturally arise. Being present is not a mental activity. Thoughts of trying to do the right thing or making plans or decisions are obstacles to this state of being. These come from a lack of trust in the value of simply being present. This lack of trust often results in a desire to control what happens, to have your own agenda and goal. Even where your goal is to help, it obscures the world of the other.

In this state of open-hearted awareness, you will share Mary's world, simply accepting and sitting with her feelings, however painful they may be. You will be sensitive to and really hear what Mary's world is like. The desire to find instant solutions, give advice or tell her what to do will not arise. Instead, you will offer her a relationship within which she can find her own way and make her own decisions. This does not mean sitting passively, doing nothing. You may well find yourself challenging Mary or asking direct questions about sensitive issues.

Self-assessment exercise 12.2
Time: 20 minutes

- Make yourself comfortable.
- Close your eyes and be still.
- Notice what arises to prevent the stillness in you.
- Notice the thoughts you have.
- Notice their nature and texture.

Awareness of what prevents you from living in the present moment is important. If you are in a state of stillness, Mary will see her reflection clearly. It is like water. Where it is agitated, the reflection becomes distorted. To offer Mary a supportive relationship, bringing loving awareness to your own suffering is important. Avoidance of your own pain and fears will lead you to close your ears and heart to her suffering. There are many ways of distancing yourself, all of which are unhelpful. One of them is to act in the role of the caring professional helper, leaving Mary in the role of the helpless. You become limited by what you think that role demands and deprive Mary of the depth and richness of who you truly are.

Your own personal journey to recognising the truth of you is fundamental to helping others. Facing your own death, loss and suffering and the mystery of life is important if you are to accompany others. It is a spiritual journey. It is not a matter of religion or knowing the answers.

Conclusion

Having faith in who you truly are and the confidence to simply be human is the key to supporting the carer. It sounds so easy but in reality it requires courage, self-searching and openness. It is more demanding than learning a set of skills. However, as human beings we have an innate capacity to love and be compassionate. It is a question of uncovering what is already there inside us all.

To learn more

- Chödrön P. *The Places That Scare You*. London: Element; 2001.
- Das LS. *Letting Go*. London: Bantam; 2004.
- De Hennezel M. *Intimate Death*. London: Warner; 2002.
- Hanh TN, *No Death, No Fear*. London: Rider; 1998.
- Kirschenbaum H, Henderson V, editors. *The Carl Rogers Reader*. London: Constable; 1990.
- Scott Peck M. *The Different Drum*. London: Arrow; 1998.

Complementary chapters

See also Stepping into Palliative Care 1: relationships and responses

- Chapter 3: The cancer journey
- Chapter 4: The experience of illness
- Chapter 5: The psychological impact of serious illness
- Chapter 6: Hope and coping strategies
- Chapter 7: The therapeutic relationship
- Chapter 15: Transcultural and ethnic issues at the end of life
- Chapter 16: Sexuality and palliative care

See also Stepping into Palliative Care 2: care and practice

- Chapter 9: The last few days of life
- Chapter 11: Breaking bad news
- Chapter 13: Spirituality and palliative care
- Chapter 14: Bereavement

Spirituality and palliative care

Stephen Wright

Pre-reading exercise 13.1
Time: 30 minutes

Sit quietly and answer the following questions about yourself. There is no need to dwell on them too deeply; in fact your immediate, spontaneous response may be the most appropriate. Ask yourself each question in turn then make just a few notes about what arises for you. Also make a note of how you feel about these questions:

1 Who am I?
2 What is the purpose of my being here?
3 Where am I going in the future?
4 How do I get there?
5 What will happen to me when I die?

- *Are they familiar to you?*
- *Did the answers come easy?*
- *Do they seem strange and difficult to respond to?*
- *Did you find yourself irritated or intrigued by them?*
- *Are they things you have thought about before or are these issues totally new to you?*
- *Are your answers different to what you expected?*

Do not worry if answers are not clear to you. The object here is to proffer a few questions that will underpin the reading which follows. For some people, the answers will be very clear and obvious if they already have well-thought out belief systems or have followed a particular faith. Thus a person who answers question 5 with 'I will be born again in another lifetime' or another who says 'I hope to go to God in heaven' is saying something about their spirituality and religion. But so too is someone who says 'I don't know'.

Is that all there is
Is that all there is
If that's all there is, my friends,
Then break out the booze
And have a ball
If that's all there is ... (Peggy Lee)[1]

Religion and spirituality

I entered nursing over 35 years ago and the emphasis of learning was very much on practical skills and body physiology, with a hint here and there of psychology or sociology as a nod to total patient care. Consideration of religious needs (spirituality was not a word in our vocabulary then) rarely got past the various dos and don'ts of the different faiths, such as whom you could and could not touch at the time of death.

We got to know the patient's religion by asking them on admission. There was a little place reserved in the top right-hand corner of the notes where Jewish, Muslim, Roman Catholic (R/C) or Church of England (C of E) could be written. Those who could not decide on their religion or did not have one somehow did not fit the rules, so they usually got labelled C of E just to make things tidy! And thus the record was complete, but largely ignored by all except the chaplains of various denominations who would visit to check which patients were theirs, or there would be a flurry of attention to it by everyone if death were looming. And that was about it.

Learning about religion and spirituality in this way was a common experience of professionals of my generation. Times have changed. Spirituality has come out of the closet of ignorance. Now debates, conferences and publications on the issue are commonplace. The shelves of bookshops groan under the weight of new-age and not-so-new-age texts giving advice on spiritual matters – everything from how to get your home more spiritual with Feng Shui to transforming your life through past-life exploration.

Self-assessment exercise 13.1
Time: 20 minutes

So, what is this thing called spirituality? Consider the following and write down half a dozen words which you associate with each:

1 spirituality
2 religion.

There is not a particular right or wrong answer. This is more concerned with your own views. For example, when I asked this question in a class recently, some participants had very clear views on spirituality as it related to the meaning and purpose of their lives. Others confused it with *spiritualism*, some thought it to be *new age* and irrelevant or irrational, and others saw it to be the same as religion. Likewise, *religion* for some people conjured up comfortable images of security in God's love, while others saw only intolerance, abuse or war associated with it.

There is much debate in the literature about definitions of spirituality and religion. For the purposes of this discussion it is suggested that everybody seeks meaning, purpose, direction and connection in life – *spirituality*. We all at some point ask questions of what it's all about and why we are here, seeking answers to all those great existential questions like *'Who am I?'*, *'Why am I here?'*, *'Where am I going?'* and *'How do I get there?'* We all pursue relationships, work and activities that nurture and feel *right* to us and imbue our lives with a sense of meaning, purpose and fulfilment of our values. For some people this pursuit is essentially God-centred, embracing the belief in some divine being(s). For others, it is essentially atheistic or at least agnostic, such as humanism or Buddhism. Our spirituality is therefore the very roots of our being – who we think we are, why we are here and what we should do with our lives, without which we can feel rootless and cast adrift, as Peggy Lee sang.[1] Religion can be seen as the ritual, liturgy, dogma and the various practices that we collectively bring to our spiritual life to codify and unify it with others. Indeed some if not most religions provide ready-made answers to those questions we ask about the nature of our being and purpose. Religion provides a channel for the expression of our spirituality. Thus, everybody is spiritual but not everybody is religious. We all seek meaning, purpose, relationship and connectedness in life, but not everybody chooses to channel that quest through the more formal structure and belief system of a religion.

When we have a health problem, we may also experience a spiritual problem. Our illness story may challenge the way we look at the world. Fears of death, loss and injury can arise. Relationships can be shaken, hopes changed, expectations adjusted. Indeed, what we feel and believe about our health can directly affect it; there is a direct impact upon our cellular structure from our emotional state[2] either positively or negatively. We therefore need to look more deeply at spirituality because it directly affects the wellbeing of patients. This in turn challenges us to find more rigorous assessment tools and more appropriate ways of addressing people's spiritual needs than ticking the religion box on the admission sheet. Furthermore, there is a growing body of evidence that stress, burnout and the disenchantment of professional carers with their work has its roots in issues more complex than pay and conditions.[3] Issues such as meaning, purpose, relationships and connectedness in work (the very stuff of spirituality) are just as important as other matters, if not more so, in producing a happy and contented workforce and an organisation that does its job well.

The spirituality revolution – are we ready for it?

There is growing evidence that a major cultural shift towards matters spiritual is taking place, in Western cultures at least.[4–8] This means that patients increasingly place different demands and expectations of spirituality in the hands of their professional. It also means that we are part of it too, for the doctor, nurse and therapist or whatever label is likely to be just as much part of this cultural shift as anybody else.

Some write of a *spirituality revolution* being under way[7,8] – a distinct trend that has been unfolding with accelerating pace in the post-war era. Within a couple of generations, an enormous cultural shift has taken place, which the sociological research supports, which has broken the traditional religion/spirituality paradigm. Religion has shrunk while spirituality has expanded. Across the board, religious allegiance has been in decline (at such a rate that if maintained by the year 2030 the congregational forms of religion will be almost extinct in the UK).[6,7] What sociologists call the *subjective turn* has drawn us away, in huge numbers, from defining ourselves in society according to external ideas of *how I should be*. On the way out is the adherence to orthodoxy, authority and absolute truth as encapsulated in the ordered pursuit of spirituality via the religions, where *who I am* is defined for me. On the way in is the rise of the personal search for meaning where the inner experience forms the new truth. The subjective turn is the turning away from finding meaning and purpose in external sources (such as the religions of *congregation* with their relatively fixed values, rules and certainties) towards the subjective personal search as evidenced in the burgeoning holistic movement.

The holistic milieu has caught professionals in its web too, for *patient-centred care* (itself a marker of the subjective turn) now lies at the centre of healthcare values. Yet for many professionals in the conventional healthcare system, largely embodied for example in the NHS, this produces conflict. Trying to make holistic, patient-centred care a reality and find personal meaning in work pushes some to the limits when constricted by the bureaucratic *iron cage* of so much of our healthcare system. This strain shows in the massive move towards the complementary therapies and the continuing exodus of staff from the conventional systems that fail to respond to the subjective turn. If professionals are themselves caught up in the subjective turn it can be a real challenge to work in an organisation that is stuck in the old paradigm where rules, targets and bureaucratic order define what should be. Indeed it could be argued that the roots of palliative care itself lie in this *subjective turn* where deep dissatisfaction arose with the dehumanisation of care of those who needed long-term care and/or were dying. The hospice movement has arisen from the milieu which began to demand more compassion, meaning and more attention to the whole person in the process of dying.

Professionals a generation or two ago formed part of that fixed order of the world. It mirrored the religious culture of the time – adherence to authority, rules, nurse (or doctor) knows best ... Now individualised care, *holistic* attention to body, mind and spirit fill our repertoire, and literature, conferences and policies urge our ever-deeper involvement on spiritual care. Front-line clinical staff and not just chaplains now find themselves asked to provide spiritual care. Urged on by professional developments and policy making (such as recent NHS papers urging more involvement of clinical staff in spiritual care[9,10]) this begs two serious questions. How well equipped are most professionals to deliver spiritual care, and what education and support do they need to do it well? Training programmes in spirituality and health are now popping up all over the place in response to the demand (and I am involved in not a few of them myself!) but is this the right way forward and can courses educate us for spirituality? I suspect the part they play may only be minor, as there cannot be any substitute for the individual commitment to ongoing spiritual practice and awakening. I suspect further that the ability to give spiritual care is directly proportional to the level of spiritual awakening of the caregiver.

Self-assessment exercise 13.2
Time: 15 minutes

Consider at this point:

- What would be your own response to a request to give spiritual care?
- Are you sure what spiritual care is at all?

It is common among professionals to feel unprepared for it, to see it as something only the chaplain should do. But reconsider this for the moment. Perhaps part of the problem comes from misunderstanding what spirituality is, as we explored at the beginning of this chapter. A certain mystique has grown up, adding to the confusion, around spiritual care being something special and unusual. Certainly, as we shall explore, effective spiritual care takes knowledge and skill, but it may be that we are already more skilful at providing spiritual care than we realise, and that to a certain degree we may be *doing it* already.

This leads to a further question. How do we discover what the patients' spiritual needs are? Spiritual assessment tools are mushrooming at the same rate as spirituality and health courses. Laudable as these efforts are, in the hands of the less spiritually mature professionals, these may well do more harm than good. A spiritually mature well-rounded human being resting comfortably in deep awareness of themselves amid all that is, armed with all the skills of their profession and of their humanity, is well placed to deliver spiritual care. Do we have enough people of this calibre and, if not, what needs to be in place to prepare and support them? At the same time it is worth considering what spiritual care is all about and not lose sight of its essential simplicity by professionalising it even further. We often give spiritual care yet do not see it as such because it has not been given that label. For example, a doctor helping a patient understand why her life has fallen apart because of drug addiction or a nurse patiently listening while a dying man expresses his anger – these are the very stuff of spiritual care, yet we may often not see it as such.

Light and shadow of spirituality in healthcare

There is quite a lot of evidence supporting the importance of spiritual care, but is there a downside as well? Much of modern healthcare seems to have lost a sense of the sacred: technically and scientifically rich, yet spiritually poor. In such a context, the spiritual needs of carers and cared for can expect scant attention. Wariness about religion, as suggested earlier; and the risks of proselytising or judgementalism creeping in coupled with an emphasis upon humanistic scientific values has led to a lack of awareness and inclusion of spirituality in healthcare. On balance, people who follow some sort of spiritual path in their lives live on average 7 to 15 years longer than those who do not. Studies on spiritual practices such as prayer and meditation point to overall health benefits.[11–13] Therefore, spirituality directly impacts upon health and wellbeing. However, some authors have expressed concern that the studies, which show such positive benefits, can be distorted by religious pressure groups to force more religion into healthcare.[14] Certainly none of the studies are conclusive that a belief in God alone will make you healthy. What seems to matter is that you believe in something – enough to give your life meaning, purpose and connection.

Furthermore there is the *nocebo* effect to consider, a reverse of the placebo[15] effect. As suggested earlier, positive feelings such as love can affect health and wellbeing for the better. However, negative ones such as depression or the feeling, among the religious, that God has abandoned or is punishing us can cause adverse health effects. This is the darker side to our spiritual beliefs. When we believe that we are not loved by God, or that God has turned against us, or, if we are atheist, simply feel hopeless, unloved and unwanted, or that there is no future for us, then we are more likely to get sick or die.

Another difficulty is the possibility of denial among healthcare practitioners that we are anything but caring and compassionate. We come into our work with all kinds of motives, some conscious and some in our unconscious.

Self-assessment exercise 13.3
Time: 20 minutes

Pause for a moment. Reflect on your own motives for your interest in palliative care.

- What makes you interested in this field and draws you to work in it?
- Have you ever worked in a setting where someone who is sick and vulnerable has been given a poor standard of care, neglected or abused?
- Who did it and why did it happen?

There is a great deal of evidence to show how professionals often fall short of their ideals. Commonly poor leadership, resources, education and teamwork are found to be significant factors. Less obvious can be what is going on inside us – our own motivations, some of them not obvious, can influence the way we treat others. For example, it is easier to talk about poor resources as the cause of a problem but more difficult to look at what is going on inside the heart and mind of the professional.

By chance in recent years I have been involved in conducting enquiries into two palliative care settings where things had gone badly wrong. I remember particularly a hospice because it made me face up to some of my own assumptions about hospice care. Surely, a setting caring for the dying would be the least likely place to let patients be neglected, abused and subject to very institutionalised patterns of *care*? There is, of course, no logical reason why a hospice should not experience problems like any other workplace, but I recognised instantly in myself that I had internalised certain beliefs about caring settings like hospices. Those assumptions were shattered when the enquiry exposed bullying and harassment of staff and failures in clinical leadership and standards of care. Many staff moved on or were disciplined or dismissed and the hospice was deeply traumatised. In this very dispiriting environment, right relationships at many levels had collapsed, and were it not for a few enlightened, indeed brave, managers and staff that sick institution would be continuing its course to this day. The place was not a complete disaster as most patients got through the system with modestly good care, but in the case of a few where it went wrong it went badly wrong, and the undercurrent of risk (e.g. not following acceptable drug error policies) was an accident waiting to happen.

The problem starts when we lose sight, for whatever reason, of the core purpose and meaning of our work. The distorted vision draws us away from reality into a world governed by our own over-inflated self-importance. We internalise false beliefs in ourselves (*we work with the dying, we are kind, we are caring*), reinforced when patients and public alike assure us of how wonderful we are, how marvellous we must be to do such a job *because I could never do it*. Even more sinister is the behaviour of some people for whom unresolved inner wounds lurking in the unconscious are acted out in the care environment[16] – compassion for others shifts into the desire to have power over them; the will to care becomes an obsession so that we neglect our own needs; the opportunity to serve becomes distorted by the need to feel needed. Such acting out from the shadowy side of our unconscious can be dangerous to both staff and patients, and the professions do not have a good track record of confronting these issues – preferring instead the comfort of denial that people who are outwardly caring can have some less than healthy motives for doing so. Spiritual practices, which we will discuss later, are one way of giving us insight into our own interior world, of healing old wounds and coming to be a more whole and well-balanced human being in the world.

Multiple checks and balances need to be in place in palliative care settings to maintain constant vigilance – such as appraisal, reflective practice, a constant questioning of values and beliefs (and, yes, this includes our spiritual practice), effective leadership, building good teams, quality-assurance programmes and so on. Otherwise, like the hospice staff I mentioned above, we can fall into the seduction of the mythology about ourselves – nurses and doctors are wonderful; *we would never do that*. The reality is that all kinds of shadowy motives lurk in individual healthcare staff.[17,18] The individual high-profile cases, such as nurses or doctors who murder, are the ones that hit the news. But there are also the less visible ill-intentioned acts which can distort caring environments into places of abuse, and there is no evidence to suggest that palliative care services are any less at risk than any other.

Providing good spiritual care

Self-assessment exercise 13.4
Time: 20 minutes

Think about the last time you had a big problem in your life, something that you perhaps found very hurtful or upsetting. If you felt unable to share this with anyone, how did this make you feel? If you did feel able to share it, how did others respond and how did their response make you feel?

When we struggle alone with some internal difficulty, the feeling that we have to manage it alone can make it more painful or make the problem seem worse. If it is all *down to me*, we can be left struggling with uncertainty about whether we are right or wrong, or get it all out of perspective, or deny ourselves access to the help we need. Telling our story to another can help us to clarify what is going on, can validate us as persons that our story is worth hearing. Conversely, we can be made to feel worse when people try officiously to help, or get emotional on our behalf, or dismiss or belittle our problem. The capacity to *listen*, and *listen deeply*, is an essential part of expert caring.

It is beyond the scope of this chapter to explore in detail the many ways we can give spiritual care and the essential factors that underpin it, but building palliative services which are *soulful* – paying attention to the spiritual needs of patients and staff – has some common and well-documented elements (for detailed summaries *see* references 11 and 18–20).

- *Soul community* of the workplace – organisations where staff feel cared for, involved in decision making and generally perceive work as *a great place to be*, where they can find meaning, purpose and connection. Staff and patients have the opportunity and are encouraged to deepen their own spiritual awareness through individual practice and collective support, e.g. through the provision of shared educational programmes, social events, reflective practice groups, access to meditation training, tai chi, complementary therapies, etc., the provision of quiet *sanctuaries* where one can experience silence and stillness.
- *Soul friends* – for patients and staff to support them in their ongoing spiritual needs and awareness. These are wise counsellors or mentors to whom we can turn for ongoing guidance when needed in our lives. They may be members of staff, and not just chaplains, who have deepened their own spiritual lives, who have walked the path before us and know how to support us in times of need.
- *Soul foods* – access in the care setting to the inspiration of poetry, music, art, nature, scripture and so on that refresh, renew and revitalise us. Work on creating 'healing environments' has been undertaken in many settings to move away from the cold and clinical approach of many healthcare settings.
- *Soul works* – developing spiritual practices which deepen our spiritual awareness and ability to help others in need, e.g. meditation, yoga, retreat time, tai chi, and so on. These can help us to stay centred and at home in ourselves, able to respond more truthfully and with integrity, able to be more mindful and fully present for others, especially if they are suffering.
- *Soul tools* – safe ways of exploring spiritual needs that are relevant and appropriate to the needs of staff and patients. These include spiritual assessment tools that can help us to discover who we are and what makes us tick. The *Enneagram*[21] is an interesting and relatively recent development of the type of personality inventory that also includes the spiritual dimension. Many settings have built on the work of Burkhardt and others[19] to develop useful tools to uncover the staff and patient spiritual needs. It is worth remembering that this is not just about questionnaire-type tools, although these can be helpful, but a spiritually mature person is needed who can make use of and transcend the limitations of questionnaires. Tools may ask questions about a person's religious beliefs, what religious or spiritual practices they follow and so on so that these can be supported by the healthcare practitioner, but will also delve into how the person copes with a crisis, how their current illness is challenging their beliefs, and what new needs are being illuminated.
- *Soul skills* – developing among staff those abilities such as the capacity to listen deeply, to be mindful and fully present for others, spiritual counselling, sensitive spiritual assessment, self-awareness and the ability to take care of one-self and so on.

Self-assessment exercise 13.5
Time: 50 minutes

Some challenging spiritual practices
Those who work for the seriously ill and dying are on the *existential edge* where caring relationships and all that is demanded as we encounter pain, suffering, loss and death can prove extremely taxing. Professionals have a long track record of helping others and knowing what is best to do, but maybe we do not always put them into practice for ourselves. For example, try doing the following and notice your reactions to them.

1 Sit quietly for 15 minutes without distractions. Pay attention to the coming and going of the breath and nothing else.

This is a simple relaxation technique which, unless you are used to it or meditation, can be really difficult. All sorts of troublesome thoughts can distract our attention. Physical, mental and emotional disturbances arise. Learning to relax and be fully present in the moment takes just that – learning.

2 Another practice that is guaranteed to press some buttons is to write your *death file* (*see* reference 11):
   a *instructions to family and friends* – telling them about them and where to find them
   b *what to do if you become incapacitated*
   c *how you want your funeral to be planned*
   d *letters to loved ones*
   e *your (living) will*
   f *all the details of your finances, etc.*

Writing a death file, planning your own funeral and exercises like this, apart from having practical results, are spiritual practices – asking us to face and resolve our own difficulties around suffering, death and dying. The process we go through in exercises like this is as important as the outcome.

3 Professionals are used to writing care plans – try writing your plan for your spiritual care:
   a *plotting out how much time you will give to it*
   b *what you will do*
   c *where you will get help, etc.*

Professionals are often poor at taking care of themselves for all kinds of reasons, yet taking good care of ourselves reinforces our essential worthiness and puts us in a far better position to care for others.

Palliative care and the spiritual practice of suffering

Reflection 13.1
Time: 20 minutes

Case scenario 13.1
Mary developed breast cancer in her late thirties, and went through mastectomy and chemotherapy and was still alive 3 years on. She told of the terrible pain, fear and anxiety she went through. But she also told of how *it wasn't all loss*. Through the support she received at the time Mary began to shift her perspective on her illness and her many relationships. She had to learn to be dependent on others, to confront her fear of dying, to rethink what was really important in her life. One thing that happened was that the illness shook her relationship with her husband, which had become stuck and dull. They broke through into new and loving depths with each other that they had not known before. She changed her job, realising that her frantic work life was less important than more time with the people she loved and pursing interests that were enjoyable to her. She also began to revisit her faith, to question her relationship with God and find renewed strength in pursuing her spiritual path once more. Mary's story is an example of how *darkness can become light*. How in suffering, fear and tragedy there can be a transformation of our way of being in the world – the very stuff of spirituality – that can in the midst of it and beyond it lead us to new depths of meaning, purpose and fulfilment in life.

What is suffering? *'Suffering is'* said the Buddha, seeing it from the grand perspective of his enlightened state as the product of the mind's interminable attachment to its fears, needs and desires. The seductive view that all suffering can be avoided is a fairly recent phenomenon, fuelled by Western scientific advances and the culture of eternal youth – the marketing of the possibility of a perfect lifestyle/body/health/home/garden, etc. Viewed from this standpoint suffering is not only resolvable but also meaningless. Yet other perspectives might see it differently. *'Suffering is grace'*, from the Hindu-influenced Ram Dass,[22] means shifting us out of our limiting view of ourselves into a deeper connection with a deeper reality. Jesus spoke of *'metanoia'* – using the suffering of this life and the things that have happened to us in the past as an opportunity to *transform* ourselves[23] and, in this case, approach God ever more closely. Suffering, from these perspectives, has meaning, purpose and possibility. Others would see suffering and how you respond to it as affecting your next incarnation – the Hindu believes that where your consciousness is at the time of God affects where you go next. Gandhi, as the gunshot hit, famously cried out *'Ram'* (God) – for to be with God in your mind at the point of death, unclouded by fear or the mist of drugs, is considered profoundly significant in spiritual evolution. For others who are agnostic or atheist, there may, as Mary's story illustrates, also be transformation in the way of being in the world – reappraising priorities, reforming relationships, redirecting life. The relief of suffering is furthermore a co-creative process (it does, after all, provide jobs for healthcare practitioners!) for we are drawn into it too. It can indeed be a tall order to see suffering as purposeful when you are in the middle of it. However, the frontier work of people like Dame Cicely Saunders and the ensuing hospice and palliative care movement, and truly holistic approaches such as that of the Bristol Cancer Help Centre, offers us practical solutions. Suffering at the end of life is neither meaningless nor inevitable. More imaginative approaches than limited drug regimes, for example, can make a reality of metanoia for all of us. Suffering can be transcended; we can be healed even while dying.

Spirituality is as much a part of palliative care as proper symptom management, but it is not a subject *out there* – something to be *done to* those who have need of us. It is a co-creative process. As we get involved in the unfolding illness story of the other, our own lives are touched. As we seek to give spiritual support to others, our own spiritual needs are awakened and must be addressed. *People in need of palliative care need well-rounded human beings – at rest in their own integrity, at one with themselves, able to be present in the moment and fully available to the other – to take care of them.* And thus we may discover in our act of caring a response to the depressing cry in Peggy Lee's song.[1] *No, that is not all there is.*

References

1   Lee P. *Is That All There Is?* Columbia Records; 1969.
2   Pert C. *Molecules of Emotion.* New York: Scribner; 1997.
3   Wright SG. Burning out and finding fire – stress, burnout and the healthcare practitioner – the approach of the Sacred Space Foundation. *Journal of Holistic Health Care.* 2005; **2**(1): 29–34.
4   Ray PH. *The Integral Culture Survey – a study of the emergence of transformational values in America.* Sausalito: America Institute of Noetic Sciences; 1996.
5   Thomas R. The I society. *The Guardian* (Archive). 1999; 17 September.
6   Bruce S. *God is Dead – secularization in the West.* Oxford: Blackwell; 2002.
7   Heelas P, Woodhead l, Seel B *et al. The Spirituality Revolution – why religion is giving way to spirituality.* Oxford: Blackwell; 2005.
8   Tacey D. *The Spirituality Revolution – the emergence of contemporary spirituality.* Hove: Brunner-Routledge; 2004.
9   National Health Service (NHS) Scotland. *Guidelines on Chaplaincy and Spiritual Care in the NHS in Scotland.* NHS HDL; 2002, p. 76.
10 National Health Service (NHS) England. *NHS Chaplaincy; meeting the religious and spiritual needs of patients and staff.* London: Department of Health; 2003.
11 Wright SG. *Reflections on Spirituality and Health.* London: Whurr; 2005.
12 Dossey L. Consciousness, spirituality and healing. *Sacred Space: the international journal of spirituality and health.* 2001; **2**(4): 8–12.
13 Coruh B, Ayele H, Pugh M *et al.* Does religious activity improve health outcomes? A critical review of the recent literature. *Explore: the journal of science and healing.* 2005; **1**(3): 186–191.
14 Sloan R, Bagiella E, Powell T. Religion, spirituality and medicine. *The Lancet* 1999; **353**(9153): 664–667.
15 Hamer D. *The God Gene.* New York: Doubleday; 2004.
16 Obholzer A, Roberts V, editors. *The Unconscious at Work.* Hove: Brunner-Routledge; 1994.
17 Snow C, Willard P. *I'm Dying to Take Care of You.* Redmond: PCB; 1989.
18 Wright SG, Sayre-Adams J. *Sacred Space – right relationship and spirituality in health care.* Edinburgh: Churchill Livingstone; 2000.
19 Burkhardt M, Jacobson M. Spirituality and health. In: Dossey B, Keegan L, Guzzetta C. *Holistic Nursing: a handbook for practice.* Gaithersburg: Aspen; 2000.
20 Wright SG. *Burnout – a spiritual crisis.* London: Nursing Standard Essential Guide, RCN Publications; 2005.
21 Riso D, Hudson R. *The Wisdom of the Enneagram.* London: Bantam; 1999.
22 Ram Dass. *Still Here.* London: Hodder and Stoughton; 2000.
23 Ross H. *Jesus Untouched by the Church – his teachings in the gospel of St Thomas.* York: Ebor; 1998.

To learn more

- Dossey L. *Healing Words*. New York: HarperCollins; 1997.
- Longaker C. *Facing Death and Finding Hope*. London: Arrow; 1998.
- Ram Dass, Gorman P. *How Can I Help*. New York: Knopf; 1990.
- Wright SG. *Reflections on Spirituality and Health*. London: Whurr; 2005.

Complementary chapters

See also Stepping into Palliative Care 1: relationships and responses

- Chapter 2: What is palliative care?
- Chapter 3: The cancer journey
- Chapter 4: The experience of illness
- Chapter 5: The psychological impact of serious illness
- Chapter 6: Hope and coping strategies
- Chapter 7: The therapeutic relationship
- Chapter 10: Understanding the needs of the palliative care team
- Chapter 11: The value of teamwork
- Chapter 12: Stress issues in palliative care
- Chapter 13: Communication: the essence of good practice, management and leadership
- Chapter 15: Transcultural and ethnic issues at the end of life
- Chapter 16: Sexuality and palliative care

See also Stepping into Palliative Care 2: care and practice

- Chapter 12: Hearing the pain of the carer
- Chapter 14: Bereavement
- Chapter 15: Complementary therapies: a therapeutic model for palliative care

Bereavement

Jenny Penson

Bereavement is a profound but common human experience. It usually refers to the loss of a loved one and it is linked to the experience of other deeply felt losses, e.g. old age, disability, trauma. Generally, our society seems to delude us into thinking that everyday life in this world is safe and predictable. Although deep down we have a dim awareness of the finite nature of our lives, we tend to live as if this was not so; as if we have limitless time ahead in which to appreciate, and work on, our close relationships.

Pre-reading exercise 14.1
Time: 25 minutes

- What have you learnt from the experience(s) of loss/being bereaved?
- How can this help you in your everyday life?
- How can it help you to reach out to others?

Take a moment to sit quietly, without distraction, and simply listen. Listen to your thoughts, your body, your being.

- What is being said to you about loss? Focus on the way in which your experiences have changed you.
- Are you a different person?
- Do you respond to another's distress differently?
- Has your own suffering enabled you to be more empathic with others?

This chapter is about *you*. It is '*you*' that you bring to your work with bereaved people. The quality of your therapeutic relationships is dependent on your '*being*' as much as in your '*doing*'. This chapter is about your reactions and feelings as well as the bereaved people you wish to help.

There are numerous perspectives on the experience of being bereaved. The best-known model is that of Elisabeth Kubler-Ross who divides her framework into five stages:

- denial
- anger
- bargaining
- depression
- acceptance.[1]

Models are useful but their limitations must be understood, e.g. never make the person fit the model. Models are signposts: guidance to possible ways forward. Most professionals use a model to inform their practice.

Key tip 14.1

Use one model until you become familiar and comfortable with it before trying another.

Self-assessment exercise 14.1
Time: 20 minutes

Here are some statements that have been made by bereaved people. Go through each one and reflect on your own experience. Note that they are not exclusive to the grief of bereavement. They are issues for anyone facing major challenge in their lives.

- What helped you?
- Are there any resources or anything anyone could have said to you that could have helped move you forward?

Write down your own reactions to each one.

- What I feel is so painful.
- I feel so alone.
- I am full of regrets.
- I don't know who I am any more.
- I feel so helpless.
- I am full of fear.
- I am very angry.

Compare your responses to Self-assessment exercise 14.1 to the following statements.

'What I feel is so painful'

Getting in touch with emotions can be frightening. The fear is of being overwhelmed, going mad, not being able to stop. Yet emotions are most usefully thought of as e-*motions*. As long as they are kept in motion, i.e. expressed, then they pass and feelings of relief and peace will follow. There is no cause to be frightened of them.

Grief has been called unattended sorrow. People attend to their painful feelings at their own pace and in their own way. They may need a safe place in which to do so.

'I feel so alone'

Loneliness is a deep-seated sense of not belonging, a need to feel part of something far greater than ourselves. Asking about spiritual beliefs may be very helpful and encouragement to explore these may help the grieving person to find meaning in what has happened.

Encouragement is needed to reach out in any way that can be managed. Suggested small steps might include going into the corner shop, going for a walk, saying good morning. Be gentle with yourself and others. Be willing to ask for help. Help another by an acknowledgement, a smile, a word – or more if and when you are able.

Many bereaved people find that they need to keep their grief hidden from the everyday world because others would not understand. Attending a support group allows them to be themselves, share their experiences and be open about their feelings and therefore can provide much comfort.

'I am full of regrets'

Regrets can cause us to *get stuck*, anchoring us in the past. When someone we love has died there is no opportunity left to make amends, sort difficulties out or to apologise for real or imagined mistakes. It may help to write a letter to the one who has died and, when written, do a ritual of some kind that involves destroying it. However, regrets may still be helpful to us in learning to behave differently in our remaining and future close relationships provided we reach a point where we can finally let them go.

'I don't know who I am any more'

Bereaved people usually experience a loss of identity. The question 'Who am I?' is one we may return to at challenging times throughout our lives. Trying to get to know yourself, as opposed to who you think you should be, may be a daunting but very worthwhile task, helping you to get in touch with your own experience. It may be helpful to encourage the taking of new steps, new experiences – however small – that can support the process of learning who you are, now you are no longer defined by the role(s) you have lost.

'I feel so helpless'

Nothing dispels helplessness more than talking about it. Our culture does not encourage the sharing of feelings; the notorious British 'stiff upper lip' still appears to be the norm particularly in healthcare. Seeking help takes courage and no more so than when the bereaved person has had the role of helper in their community.

'I am full of fear'

This breach in the security with which we get through each day can be devastating. The world is no longer predictable or safe. The need is to find security within oneself. This may encompass beliefs about God, a higher power that is in charge and in whom one can trust.

'I am very angry'

People do not always admit to anger and it may be observed rather than expressed. It may manifest as irritability over seemingly small things, or as the 'smiling anger' which masks rage with niceness. Anger directed towards oneself may manifest as guilt. Writing a letter to the person who has died can be one way of expressing negative emotions as they arise. Forgiving the person who has died – and oneself – can be the key to healing this emotion.

Self-assessment exercise 14.2
Time: 15 minutes

- What is your emotional pattern?
- Do you tend to minimise or mask your own emotional pain?
- Do you tend to exaggerate or dramatise it?
- Are you open about showing and sharing your feelings?
- Are there any changes you would like to make?

Going through the grieving process is about allowing yourself to accept your emotions as they arise, to express the pain and move beyond it. It is a cycle of change, of doors closing, of endings, of completing the past. This is followed by an uncomfortable period of mourning these losses and living with the uncertainty of what will come next. There is a need to accept this process, which is not linear but fluid.

Essentially what is needed is hope.[2] Bereaved people need to be encouraged and uplifted by those around them. They need support in trusting that restoration will come, bringing new beginnings and opening new doors. In Griffiths' model of bereavement care this is seen as resurrection after loss.[3]

The paradox is that one may be unable to enjoy life fully if one has never known deep sorrow.

> ... the most amazing thing happens. The more pain you are willing to take on, the more joy you will also begin to feel. And this is truly good news of what makes the journey ultimately so worthwhile.[4]

So far, we have explored the cognitive and feeling parts of ourselves. Bereavement is a profound experience that inevitably raises spiritual questions.

Self-assessment exercise 14.3
Time: 15 minutes

- What, if any, spiritual beliefs do you have that support you in times of trouble?
- Does God seem abstract and distant, or close and personal to you?
- Have you ever had any spiritual experiences?
- What effect did they have on you?

There is talk about meeting the spiritual needs of the people we are helping but discomfort at addressing such an intimate and personal part of the individual may get in the way.

In mental health, when it was suggested that psychiatrists take a spiritual history, they *'were amazed by what it revealed'*.[4] You may consider asking questions sensitively that elicit thoughts about belief, meaning and values that are held by the bereaved person.

The funeral service can provide a platform for people to review their beliefs and to turn or return to those they may once have held. There is a valuable opportunity for the minister who takes the service to provide comfort and lead the bereaved person into deeper explorations of loss and death, beliefs and values. Seekers who do not belong to any religious group may be helped by the Interfaith Seminary who can provide contacts with spiritual counsellors in all parts of the UK.[5]

Adopting a holistic approach means that we are concerned with the physical as well as the emotional and spiritual elements of each individual we work with. There has been far less attention in the literature to how the body experiences loss and the memories associated with it.[6] However, the growing body of knowledge from psychoneuroimmunology (PNI) demonstrates the close link between physical illness and emotional states.[7]

Self-assessment exercise 14.4
Time: 30 minutes

Take 10 minutes to be quiet. Remove all distractions and sit comfortably. Set an alarm clock if you need to. Become aware of your body. Now recall feelings of loss and/or grief.

- What do you feel?
- Where do you feel this tension in your body?
- Send warmth and love to that part of yourself, and feel it relax.

Finish this time by focusing on feeling loving and let that love spread all the way through your body.

Make it a habit to check out your body whenever you feel a strong emotion or stress. Then intentionally relax that part of you.

One holistic model of bereavement focuses on healing and renewal and includes complementary approaches to care.[8] Physical therapies, e.g. massage, aromatherapy, reflexology and healing, can help the release of deeply held pain. The intimacy of touch dissolves barriers. Relaxation and meditation with or without the use of imagery may be helpful to still body and mind and bring peace.

Emotional freedom technique (EFT) is a comparatively new psychological therapy used in the treatment of fears, phobias and negative emotions. It is reported to have been helpful in alleviating the emotional pain of bereavement. Painful memories are not forgotten but the emotional pain is discharged. While it may not be appropriate to clear these emotions at the time of the loss, they can be reduced to a manageable level. This encourages the bereaved person to share and cherish memories with others without the additional burden of intense emotional pain.[9]

Each session involves gently tapping a sequence of energy points with the fingertips, which releases painful emotions. The bereaved person can use this self-help technique whenever they need to. Case studies of EFT, used by the bereaved, are available.[10]

Self-assessment exercise 14.5
Time: 10 minutes

How can I connect with the bereaved person I am trying to help?

There are many techniques that can help us to be more fully present with those we are trying to help. These all involve various ways of calming our emotions and letting go of distractions from within or from outside us, enabling us to fully attend to the person we are with.

- *In the community*: park round the corner for a minute or two, consciously letting go of the previous visit. Then turn your attention to what you are about to do next.
- *'Softening the belly.'* We hold grief and tension in our abdomen. Drop your awareness into that area and then let it go. Blow it out a little, as if it is a balloon. This helps you to open to the moment.
- *The 'ah' breath:* involves taking on another's breath, i.e. matching the rhythm of their breathing with one's own breath can help us to *'tune in'*.[11]

Self-assessment exercise 14.6
Time: 10 minutes

- What sources of help might you suggest?

Brainstorm a list of potential sources of support and professional help.

As bereavement begins from the moment the relative knows that their loved one will not recover, support needs to start from then.

Level 1

This level is the natural support system of families and communities. Pets can be helpful, giving love and warmth, providing structure to the day and, depending on the pet, providing a means of socialising. Pets As Therapy (PAT) dogs may help animal lovers who are unable to look after pets themselves.[12]

Level 2

This level is that of volunteers and self-help groups, e.g. those run by hospices, Cruse, Compassionate Friends and churches. These legitimise and accept the bereaved person's experience, give comfort, and can provide a circle of supportive new friends.

Level 3

The level is that of the professionals, e.g. general practitioners, Macmillan/hospice nurses, counsellors, psychologists, complementary therapists, and the clergy.

Working with bereaved people requires the development of the professional skills of assessment, referral, evaluation and follow-up. Knowledge of the usual or 'normal' pattern of bereavement is necessary in order to know when the process seems to be prolonged, postponed, blocked or even excessively shortened and so further help may be needed.[13] The human skills of warmth, openness, active listening and willingness to be 'alongside' the grieving person are equally important.

It may be helpful to get across the following key points, tailoring these to the individual and his or her circumstances:

- Accept help and support when it is offered; do not turn it away.
- It is a process that takes time; do not expect too much too soon.
- Emotions need to be felt before they can be released.
- When possible, plan for the 'firsts', e.g. anniversaries, holidays.
- Surround yourself with a network of support.
- Take care of your physical health.
- Nurture hope and work on visions of a different future.

Self-assessment exercise 14.7
Time: 15 minutes

What have you learnt from challenging times in your own life that might help the recovery of others?

Recovery

Bereavement is a process, a journey towards wholeness. There are no quick fixes. Recovery happens in proportion to the significance of the loss – not overnight. Only small losses can be grieved over and healed quickly. Coming out of the wilderness takes time. Who is it that will emerge from the ashes?

Time is needed to sit with emotions in order to integrate, understand, express and ultimately heal them. Although there will be a scar forever, healing will take place. Recovery is about re-joining life and '*is not a matter of doubtless certainty but a matter of daring courage*'.[14] This is the experience of living 'on the edge', which carries with it the possibilities of new life.

The process might usefully be thought of as a kind of hibernation from which one can slowly and gently emerge, like a butterfly from its cocoon. The opportunity is to live more consciously and more fully.

The most healing thing we can do with someone in pain is to be willing to share it. The challenge is:

> ... *if they can trust you to talk about their losses ... you have helped to change the world into a better place.*[3]

References

1   Kubler-Ross E. *On Death and Dying.* London: Tavistock; 1970.
2   Penson J. A hope is not a promise: fostering hope in palliative care. *Int J of Palliative Nursing.* 2001; **6**(2): 94–98.
3   Griffiths T. *Lost and Then Found: turning life's disappointments into hidden treasures.* Carlyle: Paternoster Press; 2000.
4   Scott Peck M. *Further Along the Road Less Travelled.* London: Pocket Books, Simon and Schuster Ltd; 1997.
5   www.interfaithseminary.org.uk.
6   Hentz P. The body remembers: grieving and a circle of time. *Qualitative Health Research.* February 2002; **1**(2): 161–172.
7   Pert C. *Molecules of Emotion: why you feel the way you feel.* London: Simon and Schuster; 1998.
8   Miller B, McGown A. Bereavement: theoretical perspectives and adaptation: Canberra, Australia. *American Journal of Hospice and Palliative Care.* 1997; **14**(4): 157–177.
9   Lynch V, Lynch P. *Emotional Healing in Minutes.* London: Thorsons; 2001.
10 www.emofree.com.
11 Levine S. Mercy in the room. *American Journal of Nursing.* September 2003; **103**(9): 47.
12 www.petsastherapy.com.
13 Parkes CM. *Bereavement: studies of grief in adult life,* 3rd edition. London: Penguin; 1996.
14 Solari-Twadell PA, Schmidt Bunkers S, Wang C *et al.* The pinwheel model of bereavement. *Image.* 1995; **27**(4): 323–326.

To learn more

- B'Hahn C. *Mourning has Broken: learning from the wisdom of adversity.* Bath: Crucible Publishers; 2002.
- Klass D, Silverman PR, Nickman SL. *Continuing Bonds: new understandings of grief.* Washington: Taylor and Francis; 1996.
- Kubler-Ross E, Kessler D. *Life Lessons: how our mortality can teach us about life and living.* London: Simon and Schuster Ltd; 2001.
- Penson J, Fisher RA. *Palliative Care for People with Cancer,* 3rd edition. London: Edward Arnold; 2002.
- Penson J. Helping the bereaved and helping ourselves. In: Penson J, Fisher RA. *Palliative Care for People with Cancer,* 3rd edition. London: Edward Arnold; 2002, Chapter 12, pp. 255–268.
- *The Holy Bible*: Psalms 23, 34, 147, Isaiah 61:1, Matthew 5:4.

Complementary chapters

See also Stepping into Palliative Care 1: relationships and responses

- Chapter 3: The cancer journey
- Chapter 6: Hope and coping strategies
- Chapter 7: The therapeutic relationship

See also Stepping into Palliative Care 2: care and practice

- Chapter 1: Assessment in palliative care
- Chapter 9: The last few days of life
- Chapter 13: Spirituality and palliative care
- Chapter 15: Complementary therapies: a therapeutic model for palliative care

Complementary therapies: a therapeutic model for palliative care

Lynn Basford

Pre-reading exercise 15.1
Time: 50 minutes

1 Describe the various complementary and alternative therapies used in the context of palliative care.
2 Do you know of any clinical evidence that supports the use of complementary and alternative therapies in palliative care to alleviate pain, nausea, psychological distress and improve quality of life through the process of dying?
3 What complementary and alternative therapies are most commonly used in palliative care? Why?
4 Explore the scientific literature for the efficacy of complementary and alternative therapies used in palliative care.

Introduction

The explosive use of complementary and alternative therapies (**CAMS** – Complementary and Alternative Medical Systems) by postmodern societies to prevent, promote and restore individual health defies, at one level, reasonable logic given that there are no standards of training and education for CAMS practitioners (with the exception of osteopathy and chiropractic) that equates with professions (e.g. medicine, nursing).[1] In addition, there are questions raised regarding CAMS efficiency and effectiveness in improving and sustaining health outcomes.[2,3] However, at another level, CAMS practitioners have challenged the efficiency and effectiveness of modern medical practices, particularly in the field of palliative care.[1] Observers of these opposite views have strongly recommended the need for a balanced approach in the utilisation of modern medicine and CAMS in the pursuance of restoring not only the physical aspects of health, but an individual's mental, social and spiritual health in keeping with their traditional cultural beliefs.[4]

In 1997, Prince Charles supported the Foundation for Integrated Medicine whose overarching aims are to:

1 gather information relating to CAMS effectiveness through research inquiries
2 assess the current use of CAMS by the public and healthcare practitioners
3 support education and training and regulation

4 encourage integrative medicine through which clinical effectiveness and quality of life can be improved.[5]

These aims offer a framework through which CAMS can receive rigorous attention towards their clinical effectiveness and ensure professionals are safe and competent to practise.

CAMS defined

Complementary therapies are often associated with a distinct relationship with the mind, body, spirit, whose principal focus is to improve:

- quality of life
- psychosocial wellness
- spiritual effects of illness
- control of symptoms
- maintenance or restoration of homeostasis.

The principal philosophy is that health is multifactorial, and a multilevel phenomenon that recognises illness is associated with a disturbance of the balance between the:

- physical
- psychological
- social
- spiritual levels.

Thus, intervention is about restoring the equilibrium between all these facets while encouraging the body's own capacity to self-heal.[1] Conversely, alternative therapies are used instead of mainstream medical models, such as homeopathy and traditional Oriental medicine.[6,7] Nonetheless, alternative therapies also have an affinity with the philosophical frameworks akin to complementary therapies, thus giving them a symbiotic relationship. It is because of this symbiotic relationship that the two terms are often used interchangeably which serves to confuse rather than clarify. In addition, the evolution of language used to cluster non-conventional health therapies has added to the confusion.

In the mid-to-late 20th century the universal term used to describe unconventional therapies was *alternative*. However, when an increasing number of *alternative* therapies were used as adjuncts to mainstream medicine the term *complementary* was fostered in an attempt to better describe this integrative relationship. Currently, the literature refers to them as CAMS to denote a range of therapies within a single disciplinary framework. The Cochrane Collaboration has defined CAMS as:

> ... *a broad domain of healing resources that encompasses all health systems modalities, and practices and their accompanying theories and beliefs, other than those intrinsic to the politically dominant health systems of a particular society or culture in a given historical period, complementary therapies include all such practices and ideas self defined by their users as preventing or treating illness or promoting health and well being.*[8]

In principle, the Cochrane definition is broad. This may be seen as a useful guide but does not single out any differences between the various CAMS (*see* Box 15.1), their diverse use in clinical practice, or that they can be invasive or non-invasive. Notwithstanding, it is noted that complementary therapies are by nature very complex and defy a universal description and understanding of their therapeutic intent. In recognising this conundrum, the National Center for Complementary and Alternative Medicine (NCCAM)[9] coded CAMS into five distinct groups, with each group having similar functions:

1 *Alternative medical systems of care* – healthcare systems developed separately from Western biomedical models, e.g.
    – traditional Oriental medicine
    – Ayurvedic
    – Native American medicine
    – homeopathy
    – naturopathy.
2 *Mind–body interventions* – interventions to facilitate the mind's capacity to impact physical symptoms and body functions, e.g.
    – imagery
    – relaxation
    – meditation
    – yoga
    – music therapy
    – prayer
    – journaling
    – biofeedback
    – humour
    – tai chi
    – art therapy.
3 *Manipulative and body-based models* – based on manipulation and movement of the body, e.g.
    – chiropractic
    – manipulation
    – massage
    – reflexology
    – hydrotherapy.
4 *Biologically based treatments* – natural and biological based practices and products, e.g.
    – herbal medicine
    – enzyme therapy
    – nutritional therapy.
5 *Energy therapies* – focus on energy emanating from within the body (bio-fields) or energy coming from external sources, e.g.
    – Reiki
    – magnets
    – QiGong
    – therapeutic touch.

Box 15.1   A selection of CAMS

Acupressure	Indian head massage
Acupuncture	Magnets
Alexander technique	Massage
Applied kinesiology	Meditation
Aromatherapy	Music therapy
Art therapy	Native American medicine
Autogenic training	Naturopathy
Ayurveda	Nutritional therapy
Biofeedback	Osteopathy
Chiropractic	Oxygen therapy
Cranial osteopathy	Prayer
Environmental medicine	QiGong
Enzyme therapy	Reflexology
Healing therapies (touch; non-touch)	Reiki
Herbal medicine	Relaxation
Homeopathy	Shiatsu
Hydrotherapy	Tai Chi
Hypnosis	Therapeutic touch
Humour	Yoga
Imagery	

CAMS by public demand

Economists highlight that, globally, billions of pounds are spent annually on CAMS, which far outweighs the expenditure on conventional therapies.[5] In 2000, the Department of Health declared that one in three adults had experienced acupuncture, osteopathy, chiropractic, herbal medicine, hypnotherapy, homoeopathy, reflexology and aromatherapy. In the United States it is reported[10] that 60 million Americans used CAMS, which far exceeded visits to a primary care practitioner. It is clear there is a renaissance in popularity for the use of CAMS within healthcare that is unprecedented in modern history. Scholars claim that the use of CAMS in palliative care accounts for a large percentage of the growth pattern.[6,7] For example, it is estimated that between 7% and 64% of cancer sufferers worldwide use CAMS,[11] while in paediatric oncology the percentage is 84%.[12] Examining the characteristic nature of people using CAMS suggests that they are usually:

- more educated[13–16]
- financially more affluent[14,16–18]
- younger[7,8]
- female[7,16,20]
- treated with chemotherapy.[19]

In addition, it is contended that cancer patients use CAMS throughout all stages of the disease trajectory.[20] Scholars have further indicated that many patients needing palliative care begin using CAMS:

- shortly after their initial diagnosis when health outcomes appear uncertain
- when death is imminent.[21]

Moreover, CAMS are used because people are dissatisfied with orthodox treatments, which fail to control the progressive nature of the disease, and/or symptoms, and emotional wellbeing.[22] Professionals should be mindful that there is an increasing awareness of the relationship between health and illness that is drawn from an historical perspective,[23,24] coupled with a need for people to take control of their own health needs.[1]

Palliative nursing and CAMS

Contemporary palliative nursing practice is a complex business given the changes incurred through advancements in technology, therapeutic practices, and a plethora of research evidence. Nonetheless, the heart of nursing practice remains centred on holistic care that serves to promote health, maintain and restore health, and, when health fails, promotes a dignified and peaceful death.[1] Holistic practice requires undertaking a comprehensive assessment that considers the patient's physical, social, psychological and spiritual wellbeing: a framework that not only guides clinical practice but has an affinity with the philosophical teachings associated with CAMS. Therefore, it is clear why nursing, within the context of palliative care, should incorporate CAMS as part of everyday practice. Nursing is a therapeutic endeavour in its own right,[25] but only if there is a transfer of energy and/or an exchange of energy between the giver and receiver of care. In this sense, the process of energy transfer is through the principles of quantum mechanisms, or quantum healing.[1] Unfortunately, in the pursuit of becoming a profession, and by following the dictums of modern (reductionistic) medicine, palliative nursing practice had lost sight of its central core activity which is to provide care from a holistic perspective in the recognition that people are more than their bodily parts. Nonetheless, with the resurgence of CAMS' popularity by the public and the recognition to incorporate holism within nursing practice, the current service reforms have allowed nurses working in palliative care to assess and prescribe patients' needs from a much wider scope of therapeutic practice. However, to undertake such diverse roles and responsibilities, the nurse must demonstrate the competence to practise within the boundaries dictated by the regulatory bodies. Given the need for competence, nurses should not fear the challenge to embrace CAMS as part of their repertoire of skills as the benefits enjoyed by the nurse and patient are significant. For example, CAMS promotes reciprocal partnership so that responsibility and decision making is jointly shared. Moreover, quality of care is improved, leading to increased job satisfaction and achievement.[1]

Clinical governance and CAMS

Seeking out CAMS is a patient's prerogative, given they usually finance the service. While this appears to be an innocuous activity, it can be dangerous if used in conjunction with orthodox treatments, and, more importantly, is undisclosed to the professional. For example, herbs and vitamins are commonly taken by cancer patients with the view that they will restore health through natural processes. Little consideration is given or, indeed, known that these *innocent* properties have the potential to disguise, distort or react with orthodox therapies. Therefore, using CAMS indiscriminately as an adjunct to mainstream medicine, or as an alternative, must be avoided as it clearly creates a conundrum for the professional who, through the legal requirements of clinical governance, is held accountable. It is *important* that the professional:

- undertakes a *full* history including the patient's use of CAMS
- advises the patient of CAMS efficacy
- advises the patient of the potential dangers when used simultaneously with certain orthodox therapies.

Utilising this approach enables the professional to optimise care based on scientific and clinical effectiveness, while meeting the cultural beliefs/requests of the patient.

Self-assessment exercise 15.1
Time: 15 minutes

Consider the case scenario and answer the questions.

Case scenario 15.1

The accident and emergency unit had been particularly busy one Friday when Jane (50) presented with acute abdominal pain and distension of 24-hour duration. She had not passed wind or had a bowel movement during this period and had commenced vomiting, which was green in colour. Prior to this period Jane had complained of frequency of bowel movements for a period of 6 days. On examination her signs and symptoms were commensurate with a large bowel obstruction and she was immediately prepared for surgery. Unfortunately, the ensuing exploratory laparotomy did not disclose any obstruction, and yet the intestines were clearly grossly distended. To relieve the distension an ileotomy was performed. Perplexed by the situation the ward manager asked Jane's husband if she had been taking any alternative medication. He sheepishly said that she had taken hyoscine bromide* for her loose stools the day before the event.

Questions:
1 What is the professional's responsibility in this situation?
2 What measures should have been taken that would have appropriated correct therapeutic intervention?

(*See* answers on page 224.)

* Hyoscine butylbromide is a conventional drug used to reduce muscle spasm in the bowel.

Seeking evidence

Scientific evidence is usually determined through the rigours of randomised controlled trials (RCTs). RCTs are recognised as the gold standard, but they also have limitations when exploring the phenomena of health through a holistic perspective, as opposed to a reductionistic model. Nevertheless, in the pursuit of establishing CAMS' efficacy, CAMS practitioners have used the research methods determined by the RCT model. The Cochrane Library now cites over 5000 reports and 60 systematic reviews on CAMS.[23,26] However, there are critics who have questioned the reliability and validity of the research process used by CAMS researchers.[26] While mindful of critics' views, critiquing research findings is the norm for all scientific investigations, and should therefore not overshadow some of the emerging evidence of CAMS' efficacy. For instance, a systematic CAMS review (1966–1988), for palliative pain, dyspnoea and nausea, identified 15 studies of cancer patients who used the following CAMS:

- transcutaneous electrical nerve stimulation (TENS)
- acupuncture
- acupressure
- massage/aromatherapy
- psychosocial interventions
- reflexology
- music
- art
- hypnosis
- relaxation
- counselling
- positive coping strategies.[27]

Another review (1982–1995) demonstrated that cancer patients:

- increased their health outcomes with relaxation techniques and imagery
- reduced their pain when cognitive behavioural approaches were used.

Furthermore, reduction in pain related to cancer was effective with hypnosis and relaxation techniques.[28,29]

Self-assessment exercise 15.2
Time: 1 hour

- Explore the following websites:
  - www.cochrane.org
  - www.rccm.org.uk/Static/Links_EBM_sites.asp
  - www.compmed.umm.edu/cochrane/
  - www.nelh.nhs.uk/cochrane.asp.
- Critique the scientific evidence of one or more CAMS that is used within palliative care.

CAMS: an integrated model for palliative care practice

The complex needs of patients with cancer and chronic illness require a holistic perspective and assessment. Such an approach is at the heart of CAMS philosophy and principles that are not always centred on cure, but about supporting the health changes throughout life's continuum. In recognising the validity of an integrated model, palliative care is widening the scope of practice to embrace the use of CAMS that have a therapeutic value to the patient's health and/or improve the quality of life. In the UK, CAMS are increasingly used, and promoted, in primary care with 40% of general practices offering access to CAMS as an integrated therapeutic model.[8] Emerging evidence suggests that integrative models:

- improve quality of life
- promote the use of positive coping strategies
- control symptoms and disease progression
- encourage and improve caring partnerships with patients and their carers.[1,8]

A selection of CAMS used in palliative care

When looking at websites for an inventory of CAMS one will note that there are too many to describe each in the context of this chapter. Therefore, a selection has been chosen that represents each of the five domains described earlier.

Alternative medical systems

Traditional Oriental medicine (TOM)

TOM is not a new phenomenon; it has evolved over thousands of years and is based on Taoist philosophies and principles, dating back to 1500 BC.[30–32] According to Taoist philosophy, people maintained their health status from interacting in a dynamic way with their environment. The ultimate aim of TOM is to restore the internal balance through working with the natural life force known as Qi that moves smoothly through the body in an uninterrupted manner. According to TOM's theory, illness occurs when there is too much or too little Qi, or when the flow of Qi is blocked. In health, the flow of Qi passes through meridians (*see* Figure 15.1* – colour plate section).

Techniques

When illness presents, restoration of the flow of Qi can be restored through herbal treatment, and/or the stimulation of various meridian points through the process of acupressure or acupuncture. There are 12 major meridians and eight minor. Each of the major meridians relates to the concept of Yin and Yang that has corresponding

---

*For the meridian point abbreviations and locations visit: http://theamt.com/modules. php?name=News&file=article&sid=211. The author would like to thank AMT for the use of this diagram. Visit the AMT website (www.theamt.com) for the latest energy therapy/psychology news and information, including top articles, bookshop, free downloads, practitioner listings and events listings.

organs (*see* Box 15.1). Yin and Yang are embedded in Chinese philosophy in the recognition that the universe is compiled of opposing but complementary energy fields. When the body is dis-stressed, the balance of energy is askew; therefore, restoration of the energy balance is required. Acupressure employs a method whereby significant pressure is applied to a particular meridian point that relates to the patient's symptom/disease. Acupuncture uses the insertion of needles into the skin (no more than three inches into the surface of the skin into deep tissue) at strategic points that are left in place for about 20 minutes during which time they can be stimulated, either by hand or electrically.

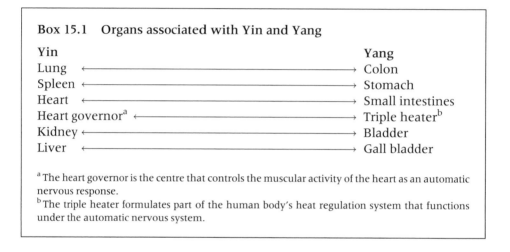

Box 15.1   Organs associated with Yin and Yang

Yin	Yang
Lung ←⟶	Colon
Spleen ←⟶	Stomach
Heart ←⟶	Small intestines
Heart governor[a] ←⟶	Triple heater[b]
Kidney ←⟶	Bladder
Liver ←⟶	Gall bladder

[a] The heart governor is the centre that controls the muscular activity of the heart as an automatic nervous response.
[b] The triple heater formulates part of the human body's heat regulation system that functions under the automatic nervous system.

Acupuncture: the evidence

Evidence of the efficacy of acupuncture has been acclaimed by the Chinese for several centuries. More recently, some studies have illustrated the effect acupuncture has on somatic and biological functioning, particularly with pain control and reducing post-operative and chemotherapy nausea, vomiting, and breathlessness.[32,33] In recognition of its common use, and to uphold standards, the United States has granted acupuncture therapists licensure status.

Mind–body interventions

Mind–body interventions are popular not only for restoring health, but as a preventative measure to sustain optimal health throughout all life's transitions.

Yoga

Yoga is an ancient Indian tradition, cited in the ancient Sanskrit *yuj,* meaning to join or unite a person's physical, emotional and spiritual wellbeing. The philosophy of yoga supports the idea that each person is connected to the universal energy and through yogic practice can achieve self-realisation and ultimate truth. In 2500 BC Patanjali wrote his treatise on yoga that described yoga in terms of eight limbs, with each limb having equal importance that together make up the whole. These are described as follows:[34]

1 Five universal commandments (yama) aimed at creating a world that is full of humanity: not harming anyone or anything; truthfulness; not stealing; leading a godly, chaste life; and not grasping.
2 Five personal disciplines (niyama): cleanliness; contentedness; self-discipline; self-study; and study of the scriptures and dedication to god.
3 Practice of postures (asana): devoted and conscientious practice of the various types of posture.
4 Practice of breath control (pranayama): practising breathing techniques with care and discrimination.
5 Detachment from worldly activities (pratyahara): developing a non-attached attitude of body and mind.
6 Concentration (dharana): being able to hold on to a subject mentally.
7 Meditation (dhyana): developing a quiet, meditative state.
8 Trance or a state of bliss (samadhi): reaching a state of absorption in a subject or in the divine.

Techniques

While there are various routes described within the yogic practices, in Western societies much attention is given to the perfecting of asanas and/or pranayama. Collectively, asanas are designed to isolate various muscle groups and organs through which the postures will both stimulate and relax. Pranayama, by contrast, is the controlling of breath, or, life force. The major effect of pranayama is considered to be therapeutic, assisting the body to self-heal and develop a strong immunity to the vagaries of ill health.

Evidence of yoga's efficacy

Through working on asanas, dharana, dhyana and pranayama, patients can:

- reduce stress levels
- restore emotional balance
- slow heart rate
- reduce blood pressure
- reduce the need for analgesia
- enable a peaceful awareness of the transition between life and death.

Furthermore, patients who have multiple sclerosis, or arthritis, can maintain joint and limb mobility.[35]

Music therapy

It has been noted that music has been associated with human activities throughout all periods in history. Music is said to enrich our souls, and is framed around life events such as weddings, funerals and celebrations. In some cultures, e.g. Native Americans, music is used to connect with the spirit world, while other cultures use music as cathartic exercise to promote psychological wellness.

Evidence of music's efficacy

Music used in palliative care can trigger emotional expression, and a review of one's life, or as a spiritual connection and a form of communication. More specifically, music can be a diversion for pain, or grief support, and improve quality of life.[36]

Meditation

Mindful meditation is primarily intended to promote relaxation and reduce distress. Its origins are rooted in religious and spiritual practices, such as Buddhist vipassana, Zen practices and yoga samadhi/pratyahara. It involves a conscious detachment and observation of the continually changing fields of our senses. Used therapeutically, it has beneficial effects. Simple meditative practice can induce a relaxation response improving health outcomes.[37]

Evidence of the efficacy of meditation

Quasi-experimental studies have demonstrated that mindful meditation can effectively reduce anxiety[38] and reduce chronic pain.[39] Other studies have demonstrated a lowering of blood pressure, lipid levels, heart rate and circulatory stress hormones. Psychologically there is marked improvement to emotional wellbeing.[40,41] One study[42] identified that cancer patients can improve or modify their coping behaviours so that they are able to pursue personal health goals and decrease mood disturbances and overall symptoms associated with high levels of stress.

Manipulative and body-based models

Massage therapy

Massage therapy has been used in a healing context since antiquity. Hippocrates was a fervent believer on the benefits of massage, particularly to induce mobility to stiffened joints. Furthermore, the Chinese and Indian communities have used some form of massage in healthcare as part of mainstream medical care for centuries. In Europe, massage did not gain recognition until the 18th century, when Dr Ling developed the Swedish Massage system to promote healing and improve lymph drainage and the body's circulatory systems.[1]

Techniques

There are many techniques applied to the art of massage. However, some common features apply that use methods of stroking, striking or kneading. Stroking (effleurage) uses sliding techniques in a rhythmical manner. It always follows the direction of venous drainage towards the heart. Striking involves using the outside edge of the hands to make short, sharp hacking movements. Striking techniques help to reduce lung congestion. Finally, kneading techniques use a firm hand pressure, moving muscle on muscle, or tissue on tissue. The kneading technique is useful for relieving tension.

Efficacy of massage

Massage improves physical and psychological health. It increases circulation and reflex activity of the central peripheral and automatic nervous system. The method of stroking increases venous return and the removal of waste products accumulated in the tissues. Psychological benefits are attributed to touch and the relaxation effect of massage. Massage can be used alone, or it can be combined with essential oils, which is then known as *aromatherapy*. Aromatherapy has many uses depending on the essential oil used. However, it is generally used to:

- promote deep relaxation
- relieve psychological distress
- reduce pain
- treat muscular conditions
- lower blood pressure
- activate the immune system
- stimulate the digestive system.[43]

In addition, massage has benefits in reducing sub-acute low back pain and promoting general improvement in wellbeing.[44]

Energy therapies

Therapeutic touch

Therapeutic touch has its roots in China and India some 5000 years ago. These cultures have recognized the concept of life energy known as *Qi* or *Prana*, respectively.[45] The ancient healer Hippocrates was known for his healing touch, as was Jesus Christ. More recently, Doris Krieger, a professor of nursing, researched the efficacy of therapeutic touch as part of a controlled trial. The results demonstrated that patients suffering from a myocardial infarction had a raised haemoglobin level, and reduced blood pressure.[1]

Techniques

Therapeutic touch is:

> ... *performed on the human energy field, which is approximately three to five centimetres beyond the skin surface. It is an effort to balance the energy field and make it uniform and smooth. This is achieved by the practitioner running her hands through the field in a head to toe direction.*[46]

Efficacy of therapeutic touch

Few RCTs have been specifically undertaken in palliative care. Nonetheless, therapeutic touch has increased the wellbeing of persons with terminal cancer.[47] In addition, therapeutic touch reduces anxiety, and acute and chronic pain.[45]

Biologically based treatments

Biologically based treatment regimes are framed around elements in nature that have a particular biological component, such as herbs, plant extracts, food nutrients and enzymes. The use of these products within healthcare can be found in the annals of history. In recent times, a search to use a biological compound in the treatment of cancer has led to many experiments. The efficacy of such compounds, as a cancer treatment, is often called into question. Therefore, the search for a cancer cure using biologically based treatments continues.

Herbs and herbal mixtures

Herbal therapy used in the context of cancer, and palliative care, predates modern medicines and chemotherapy. Their therapeutic effect has been noted throughout the process of trial and error over a long period of time. Some of these herbs have fallen on fallow ground, while others have found favour in postmodern societies for their presumed efficacy and effectiveness. Attention to herbal treatments is usually through word of mouth, or through the media, e.g. the use of mistletoe received widespread coverage after a well-known actress disclosed her use as an adjunct therapy to treat her breast cancer.

The efficacy of herbs

Mistletoe, apart from being a standard Christmas trimming having Celtic mystical powers, was used, in ancient times, by Arabian physicians.[48] It is a semi-parasitic plant member of the *Loranthaceae* family, first recommended for cancer treatment in 1916 by Rudolf Steiner. It is now marketed under various trade names within Europe. To date, the majority of the scientific scrutiny has focused on isolated compounds and whole plant extracts interchangeably. The essential essence of the herb appears to have stimulating powers on cellular function to assist in the body's immune response. However, clinical trials have not yet been able to substantiate mistletoe efficacy on cancer.[48]

Enzyme therapies

Enzyme therapies have waxed and waned in popularity throughout the modern period. In 1960, there was a revival when it was reported that tumours in mice could be prevented with oral ingested pancreatin.[49] Early human trials have suggested there is an increased survival rate with patients with adeno-carcinoma of the pancreas. Nonetheless, more robust trials are required to verify and support these claims.[50]

Oral nutrition

Adequate nutrition is the substance of life, but when there is significant weight loss due to cancer then conventional nutritional supplements do not support any nutritional benefit or weight gain.[51] Therefore, it is argued that metabolic processes that contribute to weight loss in patients with cancer may also block the accretion of lean tissue.[52] From this perspective, it is suggested that the oral administration of eicosapentaenoic acid (EPA) would stabilise the weight of patients with advanced pancreatic cancer. The study required participants to consume two cans of fish oil as a nutritional supplement each day in addition to their normal food intake. Each of these patients was losing weight at a median rate of 2.9 kg per month. After administration of the fish-oil-enriched supplement these patients had significant weight gain at 3 and 7 weeks. The patients' appetite improved and lean body mass fell significantly. The outcome of this study strongly suggests that pancreatic cancer patients who consume fish-oil-enriched supplement on a daily basis could possibly prevent cachexia.

Conclusion

Integrative therapeutic models in palliative care have increased in popularity, due in part to public pressure and increasing recognition to CAMS' contribution in:

- providing quality of life
- improved symptom management
- increased longevity
- patient satisfaction.

As with all medical treatments, it supports the clinical governance mandate if scientific evidence can substantiate CAMS use. In this sense, scrutiny of findings should inform the patient and professional, ensuring everyone is best informed of the expected health outcome and patients can be suitably informed prior to making personal choice. Given such a quest is essential, it is required that future research must seek to establish:

- CAMS' efficacy within a health context
- potential conflict when used conjointly with orthodox treatments.

When used within a palliative context, it is essential that the professional is competent to practise, thus ensuring s/he fulfils the legal requirements of professional regulation.

It is evident that CAMS are a diverse group of therapies that have been clustered together under one universal grouping. Nonetheless, they all ascribe to the notion of holism and the fact that each person has the capacity to self-heal. Vaughan[53] contends that we *take small steps each day on our journey in life, and a single step begins the journey of a thousand miles in the process of healing.* All humans have an innate capacity to self-heal through engaging with the world and the healing energies that abound. The principle purpose of CAMS is to stimulate the body's own healing mechanisms through a variety of techniques. Models of therapeutic interventions are no different from some acclaimed orthodox therapies. Therefore, we should not defer the use of CAMS until such time as there is absolute evidence given that other cultures have, through the process of clinical practice, noted the effects on all aspects of healthcare.

References

1 Basford L. Complementary therapies. In: Basford L, Slevin O, editors. *Theory and Practice of Nursing: an integrated approach to caring practice*. Cheltenham: Nelson Thornes; 2003.

2 Dipaola RS, Zhang H, Lambert GH *et al.* Clinical and biological activity of an estrogenic herbal combination (PCSPES) in prostate cancer. *New England Journal Medicine*. 1998; **339**: 785–791.

3 Lambriola D, Livingston R. Possible interactions between dietary antioxidants and chemotherapy. *Oncology*. 1999; **19**: 1003–1008.

4 White P. Complementary medicine treatment of cancer: a survey of provision. *Journal of Complementary Therapies in Medicine*. 1998; **6**: 10–13.

5 Byass R. Auditing complementary therapies in palliative care: the experience of day care massage service at Mount Edgecumbe Hospice. *Journal of Complementary Therapies in Nursing and Midwifery*. 1999; **5**: 51–60.

6 Zollman C, Vickers A. ABC of complementary medicine: complementary medicine in conventional practice. *British Medical Journal*. 1999; **319**: 901–904.

7 Zappa SB, Cassileth BR. Complementary approaches to palliative oncological care. *Journal of Nursing Care Quality*. 2003; **18**: 22–26.

8 Department of Health. *Complementary Medicine*. London: Department of Health; 2000.

9 National Centre for Complementary and Alternative Medicine. *Defining CAMS*. http://nccam.nih.gov/health/whatiscam/#2. Sourced 06–09–05.

10 Eisenberg D, Davies R, Ettner S *et al.* Trends in alternative medicine use in the national survey. *Journal of American Medical Association*. 1998; **11**: 1569–1575.

11 Ernst E, Cassileth BR. The prevalence of complementary and alternative medicine in cancer: a systematic review. *Cancer*. 1998; **83**(4): 777–782.

12 Kelly KM, Jacobson JS, Kennedy DO *et al.* Use of unconventional therapies by children with cancer at an urban medical centre. *Journal of Paediatric Haematology Oncology*. 2000; **22**: 412–426.

13 Richardson MA, Ramirez T, Palmer JL *et al.* Complementary and alternative medicine use in a comprehensive cancer center and the implications for oncology. *Journal of Clinical Oncology*. 2000; **18**: 2514–2525.

14 Lee MM, Lin SS, Wrensch MR *et al.* Alternative therapies used by women with breast cancer in four ethnic populations. *Journal of National Cancer Institute*. 2000; **92**: 42–47.

15 Burnstein HJ, Gelber S, Guadagnoli E *et al.* Use of alternative medicine by women with early stage breast cancer. *JAMA*. 1999; **340**: 1773–1739.

16 Boon H, Stewart M, Kennard M *et al.* Use of complementary and alternative medicine by breast cancer survivors in Ontario: prevalence and perceptions. *Journal of Clinical Oncology*. 2000; **18**: 2515–2521.

17 Verhoef MJ, Hagen, N, Pelletier G *et al.* Alternative therapy use in neurologic diseases. *Neurology*. 1999; **52**: 617–622.

18 Sparber A, Bauer L, Curt G *et al.* Use of complementary medicine by adult patients participating in cancer clinical trials. *Oncology Nursing Forum*. 2000; **27**: 623–630.

19 Rees R, Feigel I, Vickers A *et al.* Prevalence of complementary therapy use by women with breast cancer: a population based survey. *European Journal of Cancer*. 2000; **36**: 1359–1364.

20 Gotay C, Hara W, Issal B *et al.* Use of complementary and alternative medicine in Hawaii cancer patients. *Hawaii Medical Journal*. 1999; **58**: 94–95.

21 Sollner W, Maislinger S, DeVries A *et al.* Use of complementary and alternative medicine by cancer patients is not associated with perceived distress or poor compliance with standard treatment but with active coping behaviour. *Cancer*. 2000; **89**: 873–880.

22 Sollner W, Zingg-Schir M, Rumpold G *et al.* Attitude toward alternative therapy, compliance with standard treatment, and need for emotional support in patients with melanoma. *Journal of Dermatology*. 1997; **133**: 316–321.

23 Richardson MA, Straus SE. Complementary and alternative medicine: opportunities and challenges for cancer management research. *Seminars in Oncology*. 2002; **29**: 531–545.

24 Kelner M, Wellman B. Health care and consumer choice: medical and alternative therapies. *Social Service Medicine*. 1997; **45**: 203–212.

25 Pearson A, MacMahan R. *Nursing as Therapy*. London: Chapman and Hall; 1991.

26 MacDonald R, Mulrow C, Lau J. Seronoa repens for benign prostate hyperplasia. In: *Cochrane Collaboration, Issue 2*. Oxford: Cochrane library update software; 2000.

27   Washburn A. Complementary therapies: a survey of NCI cancer patient educators. *Cancer Practice*. 2000; **8**: 143–144.

28   Pan C, Morrison R, Ness J *et al*. Complementary and alternative medicine in the management of pain, dyspnoea and nausea and vomiting near the end of life: a systematic review. *Journal of Pain Symptom Management*. 2000; **20**: 374–387.

29   Wallace KG. Analysis of recent literature concerning relaxation and imagery interventions for cancer pain. *Cancer Nursing*. 1997; **20**: 79–87.

30   Hsu DT. Acupuncture. *Reg Anaesthesia*. 1996; **21**: 361–370 .

31   Mitchell ER. *Fighting Drug Abuse with Acupuncture*. Berkeley (CA): Pacific View Press; 1995.

32   Leake MA, Broderick J. Treatment efficacy of acupuncture: a review of the research literature. *Integrative Medicine*. 1999; **3**: 107–115.

33   Filshie J, Penn K, Ashley S, Davis CL. Acupuncture for the relief of cancer-related breathlessness. *Palliative Medicine*. 1998; **10**: 145–150.

34   Mcgilvery C, Reed J, Mehta M. *The Encyclopaedia of Aromatherapy, Massage and Yoga*. London: Acropolis Books; 1993.

35   Widdowson R. *Yoga Made Easy*. London: Hamlyn Press; 1982.

36   Krout RE. The effects of single session music therapy interventions on the observed and self reported levels of pain control, physical comfort and relaxation of hospice patients. *American Journal of Hospice and Palliative Care*. 2001; **18**: 383–390.

37   Benson H. *The Relaxation Response*. New York: Morrow; 1975.

38   Kabat-Zinn J, Massion AO, Kristeller J *et al*. Effectiveness of a mediation based stress reduction program in the treatment of anxiety disorders. *American Journal Psychiatry*. 1992; **149**: 936–943.

39   Kabat-Zinn J, Lipworth L, Burney R *et al*. Four year follow up of a mediation based program for the self-regulation of chronic pain: treatment outcomes and compliance. *Clinical Journal of Pain*. 1986; **2**: 159–173.

40   Telles S, Nagarathna HR. Automatic changes while mentally repeating two syllables: one meaningful and the other neutral. *Indian Journal Physiological Pharmacology*. 1998; **42**: 57–63.

41   Astin JA. Stress reduction through mindfulness mediation: effects on psychological symptomatology, sense of control, and spiritual exercises. *Psychotherapy Psychosomatic*. 1997; **66**: 97–106.

42   Speca M, Carlson LE, Goodey MSW *et al*. A randomized, wait list controlled clinical trial: the effect of a mindfulness meditation-based stress reduction program on mood and symptoms of stress in cancer outpatients. *Journal of Psychosomatic Medicine*. 2000; **62**: 613–622.

43   Wilkie D, Kampbell J, Cutshall S *et al*. Effects of massage on pain intensity, analgesics and quality of life with cancer pain: a pilot study of a randomized clinical trial conducted within hospice care delivery. *The Hospice Journal*. 2000; **15**: 31–53.

44   Preyde M. Effectiveness of massage therapy for sub-acute low back pain: a randomized controlled trial. *Canadian Medical Association Journal*. 2000; **162**: 1815–1820.

45   Turton P. Healing: therapeutic touch. In: Rankin-Box DF, editor. *Complementary Health Therapies: a guide for nurses and the caring profession*. London: Chapman Hall; 1992.

46   Wyatt G, Dimner S. The balance of touch. *Nursing Times*. 1998; **84**: 40–42.

47   Giasson M, Bouchard L. Effect of therapeutic touch on the well-being of persons with terminal cancer. *Journal of Holistic Nursing*. 1998; **16**: 383–398.

48   Eduard E, Schmidt K, Skeuer V. Mistletoe for cancer? A systematic review of RCT. *International Journal of Cancer*. 2003; **107**: 262–267.

49   King LS. Prevention of virus induced mammary tumours by an orally active pancreas factor. *Exp Medical Surgery*. 1065; **33**: 345–347.

50   King LS. A novel method of enhancing antibody production. *Southwest Medical*. 1967; **46**: 222–224.

51   Wigmore SJ, Ross JA, Falconer JS *et al*. The effect of polyunsaturated fatty acids on the progress of cachexia in patients with pancreatic cancer. *Nutrition*. 1997; **12**: Suppl: S27–S30.

52   Moldawer LL, Copeland EM. Pro inflammatory cytokines, nutritional support and the cachexia syndrome: interactions and therapeutic options. *Cancer*. 1997; **79**: 1828–1839.

53   Vaughan F. Human survival and consciousness evolution. In: Grof S, editor. *The Adventure of Self-Discovery, dimensions of consciousness and new perspectives in psychotherapy and inner exploration*. Albany: State University of New York Press; 1988.

To learn more

- Basford L. Complementary therapies. In: Basford L, Slevin O, editors. *Theory and Practice of Nursing: an integrated approach to caring practice*. Cheltenham: Nelson Thornes; 2003, Chapter 31, pp. 569–596.
- Peters D, Chaitow L, Morrison S *et al. Integrating Complementary Therapies in Primary Care: a practical guide for health professionals*. Edinburgh: Churchill Livingstone; 2001.
- Rankin-Box DF. *Complementary Health Therapies: a guide for nurses and the caring profession*. London: Chapman Hall; 1992.
- Harvey D. *The Power to Heal: an investigation of healing and the healing experience*. Wellingborough, Nottingham: Aquarian Press; 1983.

Complementary chapters

See also Stepping into Palliative Care 1: relationships and responses

- Chapter 2: What is palliative care?
- Chapter 3: The cancer journey
- Chapter 4: The experience of illness
- Chapter 5: The psychological impact of serious illness
- Chapter 7: The therapeutic relationship
- Chapter 11: The value of teamwork
- Chapter 12: Stress issues in palliative care
- Chapter 15: Transcultural and ethnic issues at the end of life

See also Stepping into Palliative Care 2: care and practice

- Chapter 1: Assessment in palliative care
- Chapter 13: Spirituality and palliative care

Answers to Self-assessment exercise 15.1

1 The professional's responsibility is to ensure that s/he has endeavoured to seek out all therapeutic activities the patient has engaged in during this episodic illness.
2 A holistic and comprehensive assessment should have been undertaken, which in this instance would have:
  a prevented unnecessary surgery or
  b resulted in less radical surgery.

Chapter 16

The special needs of the neurological patient

David Oliver

Pre-reading exercise 16.1
Time: 15 minutes

Before reading this chapter, consider the following question.

- How does the palliative care of a patient with a progressive neurological disease differ from that of a patient with cancer?

Test your knowledge again when you have reached the end of the chapter.

Introduction

Many chronic neurological diseases have no curative treatment. Therefore, the aim from the time of diagnosis is to provide palliative care. There are specific symptom management needs for each disease process, but the overall palliative care approach will be similar for all patients, regardless of diagnosis. However, there may be differences in approach compared to the palliative care of a person with advanced cancer. The chapter aims to explore some factors that should be taken into account when caring for a patient with a neurological disease. Motor neurone disease (amyotrophic lateral sclerosis) is used as an example to demonstrate some of these differences.

Diagnosis

Motor neurone disease (MND), like many neurological diseases, is uncommon. Symptoms may be present for some time before diagnosis is clear. This may be difficult for the patient and family. The aim is to provide support at this time and to facilitate the investigations and results so that the period of uncertainty is minimised. Delays may cause different emotions, ranging from anger, frustration and/or denial. Time may be needed to allow the patient and family to talk about their feelings. Encouragement of discussion, explanation, and expression of feelings can facilitate coping strategies for families with a progressive illness.

As the diagnosis becomes clear, and the patient and family are informed, increased provision of support and listening is important. However, of equal importance is to permit the patient's own space.[1] The patient and family should be encouraged to ask about the disease and the management. Coordination with the neurological services is essential. Many neurological centres have specialist nurses who will be with the patient and family at this time and who can listen, provide support and answer questions. Patients are often unable to absorb all that is said. Therefore, information needs ongoing repetition to ensure clarity. The specialist nurse may need to liaise with the community services so that the care plan is clear, and to facilitate effective information gathering for the patient and family.[2]

Case scenario 16.1 (part 1)

Mr C, a 60-year-old man, was married with two sons, aged 25 and 28, living at home. He had developed problems with muscle cramps in his legs and then a foot drop. He started to limp and tended to fall over when dressing as his balance was poor. He noticed that his hand movements were affected and he was unable to count money. He saw his GP and was referred to a neurologist. Following hospital investigation, 13 months after he first noticed the limp, MND was diagnosed.

Even after diagnosis, the patient and family may have little knowledge of the disease. MND is a rare disease (5000 UK patients). Few people have had contact with someone with the disease, whereas most individuals have known someone with cancer and have some idea of possible disease progression. Unfortunately, many individuals hear of MND from the press reports of court hearings of people asking for the right to assisted suicide or euthanasia, e.g. Diane Pretty who asked the courts for permission for her husband to assist in her suicide and talked of her fears of choking and suffering a distressing death. Although this is rare, with good palliative care, the message of 'distress' remains in many people's minds. Therefore, it is important to permit the patient to obtain accurate information. Voluntary associations and societies, such as the Motor Neurone Disease Association, can provide information, leaflets and help. Many areas have support groups or advisors who can visit patients and families at home.

The role at the time of diagnosis includes:

- *listening*
- *supporting*
- *facilitating* investigations and results
- *information* from neurology services and voluntary associations
- *encouraging* communication.

Disease progression

After the initial shock of the diagnosis, patients and families may need some time to acknowledge and discuss the effects on their lives. There is often no curative treatment for a neurological disease. At best, treatment may reduce the speed of deterioration and/or the effects of the disease on the patient. Although MND has no curative treatment, the drug riluzole (Rilutek – 50 mg twice a day – blocks the action of the neurotransmitter glutamate within the brain) has been shown to extend life for several months. However, it is not a cure and there will be later deterioration. Then, the care will be palliative, aiming to ensure that the quality of life is as high as possible.[3]

Initially, the patient and family may face losses, some small, and some larger. With MND, there may be loss of movement of the arms or legs, or a reduction in speech or swallowing. Moreover, there are other subsequent losses of mobility, ability to continue in employment, and/or communication difficulties. Some losses are less visible, e.g.:

- loss of role within the family
- loss of status
- loss of friendships.

There may be many small losses, which add up in time to an increasing disability and restriction on the patient's lifestyle. The aim at this time is to support the patient and family through the losses, and to ensure that careful assessment is made of the patient's abilities and needs[3] (*see* Box 16.1).

Box 16.1   Disciplines involved in coordinated care

- Nurses – specialist neurology nurse, specialist palliative care, e.g. Macmillan nurse, community nurse.
- Medical staff – consultant neurologist, rehabilitation consultant, palliative medicine consultant.
- Physiotherapist.
- Occupational therapist – hospital and social services.
- Social worker.
- Clinical psychologists.
- Counsellor.
- Bereavement counsellor.
- Family support team.
- Speech and language therapist.
- Dietician.
- Chaplain/religious leader.
- Voluntary support agencies, e.g. MND Association.
- Social services care manager.

Specialist palliative care services are able to help in this interdisciplinary assessment of patients, especially with MND, and prefer to get to know the patient and family during the early stage of the disease, while verbal communication is retained or not too greatly affected.

Careful assessment of all aspects of the patient's problems is essential, and is summarised below.

Physical aspects

These include the following:

- positioning
- pain
- dyspnoea
- dysphagia
- muscle stiffness
- communication difficulties
- constipation
- oedema.

Positioning

With increasing muscle weakness, it may become difficult to find a comfortable position. Careful assessment to ascertain the best position for the patient is necessary ensuring comfort is maintained.

Pain

Although the sensory nerves are not affected in MND, over 70% of patients complain of pain.[4,5] This may be due to muscle cramps, joint discomfort due to abnormal muscle tone around the joint, or skin pressure pain resulting from immobility. The correct treatment can be given after assessment, e.g.:

- *cramp*: muscle relaxants
- *joint pain*: non-steroidal anti-inflammatory drugs (NSAIDs)
- *skin pressure*: analgesics (including opioids).[5,6]

Physiotherapy may be helpful for maintaining all available movement and reducing discomfort and contractures in all of the above.

Dyspnoea

With increasing intercostal and diaphragmatic muscle weakness, breathlessness may occur. It is essential that professionals remain relaxed to reduce any anxiety that may exacerbate the dyspnoea. Opioid medication can be very helpful[5,6] and consideration may be given to ventilatory support,[7] which can be helpful in the relief of symptoms from chronic ventilatory failure at night. Commonly these patients sleep badly and may:

- experience nightmares
- feel unwell
- have headaches in the morning
- have change in personality
- have reduced appetite.[7]

Non-invasive ventilation, using a face mask, can be helpful. However, there is a risk that this can progress to full invasive ventilation, with a tracheostomy, if there is insufficient preparation and discussion about the future, and plans to cope with increasing dyspnoea as the disease progresses. The disease will still progress and there is a risk of the patient becoming 'locked in' with no form of communication. There are then ethical debates, as to whether ventilation should be continued, which are extremely difficult for all concerned.[8]

Case scenario 16.1 (part 2)

In the 6 months following his diagnosis, Mr C became weaker and he required new aids at home, including a banister on the stairs, a splint for his foot and a walking stick. His speech became slurred and, on occasions, he spluttered with food.

He complained that he was getting up to pass urine several times a night and was sleeping badly. He was waking in the night, felt breathless at times, woke with a headache and was not eating well. Investigations showed that he was in respiratory failure and non-invasive ventilation was commenced. He slept well, felt better, was more alert during the day, and his appetite had improved.

Dysphagia

An assessment by a speech and language therapist is supportive in planning the management of swallowing difficulties. Careful feeding and alteration of food consistency to aid swallowing can be helpful. A percutaneous endoscopic gastrostomy (PEG) or radiologically inserted gastrostomy (RIG) may be considered, and can be beneficial in reducing the stress of feeding.[9,10] A dietician will be helpful in these discussions and referral should be early in the disease progression.

Self-assessment exercise 16.1
Time: 20 minutes

- Imagine a *real incident* that has influenced *your* life, e.g. you have just got the best job, you have found that perfect partner, the house has fallen down! Now imagine if you could *not communicate* that to others. What influences would this have on:
  - you
  - your family
  - your friends
  - your work colleagues
  - your carer
  - your care.
- What would have helped you *communicate* your needs or news to others?

Case scenario 16.1 (part 3)

Six months later, Mr C was having increasing problems swallowing. Meals were taking a long time to finish. He did not '*want to be kept going*' but wanted to remain at home. After many discussions, a radiologically inserted gastrostomy (RIG) was arranged. Within a few weeks, he was requiring most of his nutrition from enteral feeding, using the RIG.

Communication difficulties

Speech may be affected if the innervation of the head, neck and respiratory muscles becomes affected. Speech may initially sound slurred but may deteriorate greatly, becoming unintelligible due to oral muscle weakness.

It is essential to listen carefully to the patient, allowing sufficient time to speak without interrupting or finishing sentences. The speech and language therapist will assess and advise on communication difficulties. Aids may become necessary, e.g.:

- *simple aids* – a pad and pencil
- *small portable aids* – a Lightwriter
- *complex computer systems.*

The care team should be familiar with these aids. It is important to ask the patient one question at a time allowing time to communicate and/or use these alternative communication systems.[11]

Other symptoms

These may include:

- constipation
- anxiety
- depression
- hunger
- muscle stiffness.

All require careful multidisciplinary involvement.[12] It is, therefore, essential that the team meet regularly to coordinate care and equipment. To avoid confusion, it is important to ensure that the numbers of professionals visiting do not overwhelm the patient and family.

Psychosocial aspects

These include:

- diagnosis
- prognosis
- physical and mental changes
- fears

- progression
- sexuality.

Patients and family facing a progressive neurological disease have fears, anxieties and concerns,[13] which may include:

- *The disease* – people may know little and read misleading information in health-related books.
- *The disease progression* – fears about the disease and becoming disabled and dependent.
- *The prognosis* – fears about the prognosis, process of dying or death itself.
- *Other physical or mental changes* – there may be fears of mental deterioration. Unlike in some neurological conditions (e.g. dementia in multiple sclerosis and Huntington's disease), in MND confusion is rare (less than 10%). However, evidence of frontal lobe damage is increasing, which may explain the problems encountered by patients in making decisions about care and the personality change that may be seen.
- *Sexuality* – patients and the families may find it difficult to discuss these issues. However, studies suggest that if the professional is willing to talk about sexuality, without embarrassment, patients have many concerns to discuss.[13] In MND, sexual function is usually unaffected, but couples may need advice and permission to cope with the difficulties and changes that occur due to increasing disability. Advice on the use of positions and/or mutual masturbation may be helpful. One patient in a survey of sexuality and MND wrote 'thank God *that* isn't a muscle' and described how helpful it had been that a nurse had discussed sexuality with him and his partner, as a couple, and encouraged experimentation and continuation with the sexual aspect of their relationship.

The family is important

The family of patients with a neurological illness need support, advice and help.[14] They have their own concerns, which may be different from those of the patient.

- *Fear of the illness* – families have their own fears of the illness, e.g. families of patients with MND often fear the terminal stages of disease progression, or developing the disease themselves. For a small number this may be a real concern with familial MND (5–10% of all people with MND), or with other neurological illnesses with a known genetic basis, e.g. Huntington's disease.
- *Communication difficulties* – patients with a neurological illness may experience particular communication problems, as the motor speech mechanisms can be affected by the disease process. These range from:
  - changes in the brain, e.g. a cerebral tumour, causing alteration in the patient's language or word-finding abilities (dysphasia)
  - difficulties caused by weakness of the muscles of the head and neck, e.g. bulbar palsy of MND
  - mental deterioration – affects the ability to communicate, e.g. dementia.
  Support of the patient and family is essential when coping with these difficulties. The wider interdisciplinary team approach is helpful. Involving the speech and language therapist at an early stage in assessing and maintaining communication skills is essential. Communication aids, e.g. spelling board or sophisticated

computer systems, may be beneficial helping a patient and family to continue to communicate.[11] There may be communication difficulties within the family, and support and encouragement in sharing feelings together may be needed. Facilitation by the professional can be helpful.[14]

- *Finance* – the care of a severely disabled person may necessitate the spouse or partner leaving employment, and financial problems can ensue. Referral and advice from a social worker or care manager may help to reduce financial stresses.
- *Children* – families attempt to protect children and grandchildren from distress by excluding involvement with the patient and the disease. Children (of all ages) realise that 'all is not well', although the extent of the knowledge depends on their age, maturity and previous experiences. Families should be actively encouraged to include the children. The help and advice of a social worker is invaluable in helping parents and the children to talk about the illness and the future. Informing and involving the school is helpful, so that everyone is aware of possible stresses on the children.
- *Difficult decisions* – families encounter difficult decisions when someone has a neurological illness. These include decisions about continuing or ending treatment regimes, e.g. enteral feeding or ventilation. Support is essential. Although the ideal may be for the patient and family to be involved in the decision-making process, this may not always be possible. There may be conflict between the views of the patient and family, or different members of the family. Therefore, close involvement and discussion with families is important. Families should be involved and included in decision-making processes, without experiencing the burden of being the only ones to make the decision.

Key workers and the wider interdisciplinary care team need to be open to the concerns of the patient and family. Listening carefully to what concerns them. Never *assuming* what is affecting them. A social worker or family counsellor is particularly effective in helping a patient and family cope with the changes and fears.

Spiritual aspects

Patients may have concerns of a spiritual nature, e.g., asking '*why me?*' or '*what is going to happen to me when I die?*'. Listening is essential – never use a dogmatic approach. There are no easy answers. Time spent listening to the patient and sharing their concerns may be sufficient. However, specialised help from, for example, a religious leader, psychologist, social worker or counsellor should be invoked promptly when indicated.

Disease progression

Assessment as the disease progresses includes:

- listening
- intra- and interdisciplinary coordinated care
- involving the patient and family

- assessment and relief of symptoms
- physical, psychological, social and spiritual care.

Specialist palliative care services may become involved in the care of patients during the early stages of the disease, or as deterioration occurs.[3]

- *Advice and support at home* – of the specialist interdisciplinary team is helpful in the care of the patient and family.
- *Hospice day therapy* – permits family respite, interdisciplinary assessment, socialisation for the patient and specific help, e.g. physiotherapy or occupational therapy.
- *Inpatient care* – permits interdisciplinary assessment of symptoms, family respite and/or for the terminal stages.
- *Hospital palliative care team* – provide advice and support in hospital.

The terminal stages

During this time, the patient may be able to fulfil personal aims and prepare for the future. This could include:

- visiting friends or family
- making a will
- organising the funeral
- preparing audio-tapes or letters for children or grandchildren
- ensuring that all of the family finances are sorted out
- helping family and friends with the grief they may be feeling
- planning further care, e.g. considering possible admission to a nursing home or a hospice.

These may be difficult activities for some patients. Encouragement to start or complete them may be needed, and the carer has an important role in encouraging the patient and family to make the most of the time they have left together. It is important the patient remains as active as possible and continues to be involved in the care and decisions that may have to be made.

Case scenario 16.1 (part 4)

Three months later Mr C's condition had deteriorated. He remained at home but was now very weak and needing increasing care. He communicated using a Lightwriter. He received his feeds via the RIG. He was distressed at times. He felt frustrated and expressed concerns that he did not want to be kept alive, or to have any treatment that would prolong his life. He received morphine to ease his dyspnoea, together with sublingual lorazepam when he became anxious. He died peacefully at home.

Professionals should be prepared as deterioration occurs. At this time, it is important that the team discuss plans, particularly the following:

- *Place of care* – will the patient be able to remain at home, or should admission to a hospice or hospital be considered?
- *Extra help* – is 24-hour care from social services or nursing care indicated?
- *Available medication* – should medication be provided so that it is available if necessary?
- *Family need* – what might be needed? How can this be accommodated?

Many patients with MND fear choking and dyspnoea in the terminal stages of the disease. With good symptom management, this should not be a problem. Studies have confirmed that death is not distressing for most patients.[5,15]

Breathing space kit

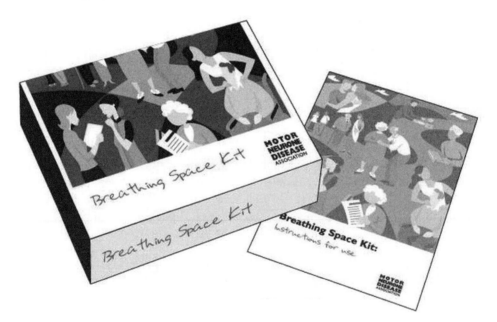

Figure 16.1   The Breathing Space Kit.
(Reproduced with the kind permission of the Motor Neurone Disease Association)

The MND Association produced a '*Breathing Space Kit*' to help to reassure patients and families (*see* Figure 16.1). The kit consists of a:

- *leaflet* – on the care that may be necessary in the terminal stages, including a discussion on medication that may be required
- *box* – to hold medication.

After discussion between the patient, family, doctor and nurse, the medication can be provided as follows:

- *for analgesia* – diamorphine 5–10 mg (or according to the oral dose)
- *for sedation* – midazolam 5–10 mg

- *to reduce secretions* – glycopyrronium bromide 200 micrograms or hyoscine hydrobromide 400 micrograms.

If there is a possibility of delayed contact by professionals providing help in an emergency, it could be suggested to the family that they give a *buccal* preparation of *midazolam* to relieve anxiety and panic, while awaiting help.

The medication stored in the Breathing Space Kit box is available in the event of a crisis, and can be administered by the professional visiting the patient, and should help the professional understand what has been discussed, and agreed, by the patient and family. If the patient subsequently improves, the return to oral medication may be possible. Alternatively, a continuous subcutaneous infusion administered by syringe driver may be considered. The presence of the kit may provide reassurance and security for both the patient and family.

Other medication may be necessary to manage symptoms:

- *analgesics* – for pain and dyspnoea
- *muscle relaxants* – for spasm
- *anticholinergics (e.g. hyoscine)* – for chestiness
- *anticonvulsants* – to prevent fits.

It may be possible to give this medication orally until near to death.[5,12,15] However, parenteral medication may become necessary, given by regular subcutaneous or intramuscular injection or continuous subcutaneous infusion by syringe driver.

Bereavement

The care of the family in bereavement starts before the death, as the care of the patient and family throughout the disease progression will influence the bereavement. Encouragement to express feelings between the family members helps the grieving process. The carer needs to be available to answer any questions the family has about the death, and support them.

During long periods of caring for a patient with a slowly progressive disease, feelings of relief from the strain of caring, mixed with guilt at these feelings, need to be acknowledged and carefully managed.[16] Many families can work through these feelings with the support of other family members and friends. However, others may benefit from professional management from the general practitioner, a counsellor, psychologist, social worker or psychiatrist.

Essential intra- and interdisciplinary approach

As the patient's condition deteriorates, there is a need to ensure that symptoms are controlled as effectively as possible, and concerns of the patient and family are addressed. Individuals involved in the care of the patient should be aware of any deterioration, and communicate any concerns. Often, some team members do not appreciate the change in care. This leads to confusion in care aims that in turn leads to confusion and loss of faith in the caring team.

The involvement of the specialist palliative care intra- and interdisciplinary team facilitates patient and family care. Other teams may be involved, including the specialist neurology team, disability team and voluntary groups, e.g. MND Association (*see* Box 16.1). Therefore, it is essential that there is coordination, and the primary healthcare team plays an important role in ensuring that continuity of care is collaborative.

Coordinating care

With so many professionals involved in the care of the patient and family (*see* Box 16.1 on page 227), it is essential to have regular coordinating care meetings. A 'key worker' ensures that care is coordinated. This prevents the patient and family being overwhelmed and disconnected from care provision. In order to maintain independence and control, the patient and family must feel supported and understood. As the patient and family's needs continually change, the primary worker must change.

Conclusion

With a coordinated approach, the progression of MND can be effectively managed for the patient and family, and the fear and anxieties addressed promptly and appropriately. The aim is to provide psychological support, and medical intervention, to a high quality standard, matching the need for intervention with the need of the individual receiving that intervention.

Self-assessment exercise 16.2
Time: 10 minutes

1 Specialist palliative care services may be involved in the palliative care of a patient with a progressive neurological disease:
   a early in the disease process
   b only if there are severe symptoms
   c only in the terminal stages of the disease
   d if the neurologist insists on their involvement.

2 A percutaneous endoscopic gastrostomy may be suggested:
   a only if there are severe swallowing problems, in the final stages
   b early in the disease process, before there are appreciable problems with swallowing
   c when swallowing is starting to be difficult and the patient is losing weight
   d when swallowing is difficult and meals are becoming a problem.

3 In a crisis when the patient is distressed with their breathing:
   a a doctor should be called and antibiotics given
   b the patient should be turned on their side and suction given
   c an injection of diamorphine with midazolam and glycopyrronium or hyoscine should be given
   d the patient's family should be excluded from the room so that they do not become further distressed by the situation.

---

4 When assessing a patient, the sexual needs of the patient and partner:
   a should rarely be a problem if they are over 60 years of age
   b rarely present a problem as the disability progresses
   c should be addressed sensitively with all couples, regardless of age
   d should only be considered if the patient is in a stable heterosexual relationship.

5 Pain:
   a never occurs in MND as the sensory nerves are unaffected
   b may be relieved by opioids, especially if there is general discomfort
   c may be related to muscle spasm
   d is usually due to some other cause and not MND.

(*See* answers on page 238.)

References

1 Borasio DG, Sloan R, Pongratz D. Breaking the news. In: Oliver D, Borasio GD, Walsh D, editors. *Palliative Care in Amyotrophic Lateral Sclerosis*. Oxford: Oxford University Press; 2000.
2 O'Brien MR. Information-seeking behaviour among people with motor neurone disease. *Br J Nursing*. 2004; **13**(16): 964–968.
3 Oliver D. Palliative care. In: Oliver D, Borasio GD, Walsh D, editors. *Palliative Care in Amyotrophic Lateral Sclerosis*. Oxford: Oxford University Press; 2000.
4 Oliver D. The quality of cure and symptom control – the effects on the terminal phase of ALS/MND. *J Neurol Sci*. 1996; **139**(Suppl.): 134–136.
5 O'Brien T, Kelly M, Saunders C. Motor neurone disease: a hospice perspective. *BMJ*. 1992; **304**: 471–473.
6 Oliver D. Opioid medication in the palliative care of motor neurone disease. *Palliative Med*. 1998; **12**: 113–115.
7 Lyall R, Moxham J, Leigh N. Dyspnoea In: Oliver D, Borasio GD, Walsh D, editors. *Palliative Care in Amyotrophic Lateral Sclerosis*. Oxford: Oxford University Press; 2000.
8 Oliver D. Ventilation in motor neuron disease; difficult decisions in difficult circumstances. *Amyotroph Lateral Scler Other Motor Neuron Disord*. 2004; **5**: 6–8.
9 Wagner-Sonntag E, Allison S, Oliver D *et al*. Dysphagia In: Oliver D, Borasio GD, Walsh D, editors. *Palliative Care in Amyotrophic Lateral Sclerosis*. Oxford: Oxford University Press; 2000.
10 Hefferman C, Jenkinson C, Holmes T *et al*. Nutritional management in MND/ALS patients: an evidence based review. *Amyotroph Lateral Scler Other Motor Neuron Disord*. 2004; **5**: 72–83.
11 Scott A, Foulsom M. Speech and language therapy In: Oliver D, Borasio GD, Walsh D, editors. *Palliative Care in Amyotrophic Lateral Sclerosis*. Oxford: Oxford University Press; 2000
12 Borasio GD, Oliver D. The control of other symptoms In: Oliver D, Borasio GD, Walsh D, editors. *Palliative Care in Amyotrophic Lateral Sclerosis*. Oxford: Oxford University Press; 2000.
13 Wasner M, Bold U, Vollmer TC, Borasio GD. Sexuality in patients with amyotrophic lateral sclerosis and their partners. *J Neurol*. 2004; **251**: 445–448.
14 Gallagher D, Monroe B. Psychosocial care. In: Oliver D, Borasio GD, Walsh D, editors. *Palliative Care in Amyotrophic Lateral Sclerosis*. Oxford: Oxford University Press; 2000.
15 Neudert C, Oliver D, Wasner M, Borasio GD. The course of the terminal phase in patients with amyotrophic lateral sclerosis. *J Neurol*. 2001; **248**: 612–616.
16 McMurray A. Bereavement. In: Oliver D, Borasio GD, Walsh D, editors: *Palliative Care in Amyotrophic Lateral Sclerosis*. Oxford: Oxford University Press; 2000.

To learn more

- Beresford S. *Motor Neurone Disease*. London: Chapman and Hall; 1995.
- Leigh PN, Abrahams S, Al-Chalabi A *et al*. The management of motor neurone disease. *Journal of Neurology, Neurosurgery and Psychiatry*. 2003; **74**(Suppl IV): iv 32–iv 47.
- Neilson S, Clifford Rose F. *Motor Neuron Disease – the 'at your fingertips' guide*. London: Class Publishing; 2003
- Oliver D. *Motor Neurone Disease*, 2nd edition. London: Royal College of General Practitioners; 1994.
- Oliver D. *Motor Neurone Disease: a family affair*, 2nd edition. London: Sheldon Press; 2002.
- Oliver D, Borasio GD, Walsh D, editors. *Palliative Care in Amyotrophic Lateral Sclerosis*. Oxford: Oxford University Press; 2000.
- Voltz R, Borasio GD, Bernat J, Maddocks I, Oliver D, Portenoy RK, editors. *Palliative Care in Neurology*. Oxford: Oxford University Press; 2004.

Complementary chapters

See also Stepping into Palliative Care 1: relationships and responses

- Chapter 2: What is palliative care?
- Chapter 4: The experience of illness
- Chapter 5: The psychological impact of serious illness
- Chapter 12: Hearing the pain of the carer
- Chapter 13: Communication: the essence of good practice, management and leadership
- Chapter 14: Ethical dilemmas
- Chapter 16: Sexuality and palliative care

See also Stepping into Palliative Care 2: care and practice

- Chapter 9: The last few days of life
- Chapter 13: Spirituality and palliative care
- Chapter 14: Bereavement

Answers to Self-assessment exercise 16.2

1 a.
2 d.
3 c.
4 c.
5 b and c.

Useful contacts

Alzheimer's Disease Society
Gordon House, 10 Greencoat Place, London SW1P 1PH
General enquiries: 020 7306 0606
Helpline: 08453 000 336 (8:30 am to 6:30 pm, Monday to Friday)
Email: info@alzheimers.org.uk
Website: www.alzheimers.org.uk

The Alzheimer's Disease Society is a care and research charity for people with Alzheimer's disease and other forms of dementia, their families and carers. It is a national membership organisation and works through nearly 300 branches and support groups. There is a wealth of information available on the website including fact and advice sheets.

Bereavement Research Forum
Bereavement Research Forum Administrator, Bereavement Service
St Joseph's Hospice, Mare Street, Hackney, London E8 4SA
Tel: 020 8525 6031
Email: s.cornford@stjh.org.uk
Website: www.brforum.org.uk

The Bereavement Research Forum provides opportunities for the discussion and development of bereavement research and the promotion of research into policy and practice. Three symposia are held annually and a conference every other year. The website gives further information about the organisation, membership and activities.

Breast Cancer Care
Kiln House, 210 New Kings Road, London SW6 4NZ
Tel: 020 7384 2984
Helpline: 0808 800 6000 (9 am to 5 pm, Monday to Friday; 9 am to 2 pm, Saturday)
Fax: 020 7384 3387
Email: info@breastcancercare.org.uk
Website: www.breastcancercare.org.uk

Breast Cancer Care offers practical advice, information and support to women concerned about breast cancer. Its services include a wide range of booklets, leaflets and audiotapes, a prosthesis-fitting service and one-to-one emotional support from volunteers who have experienced breast cancer. BCC aims to help anyone who needs its services – women with breast cancer, with other breast-related problems or who are worried about their breast health, families, partners and friends, members of the general public who need information, doctors, nurses and other health professionals, and the media.

Bristol Cancer Help Centre
Grove House, Cornwallis Grove, Bristol BS8 4PG
Reception: 01179 809 500
Helpline: 08451 232 310 (9:30 am to 5 pm weekdays or 24-hour answerphone)
Email: info@bristolcancerhelp.org ; Helpline@bristolcancerhelp.org
Website: www.bristolcancerhelp.org

Bristol Cancer Help Centre is the holistic charity that pioneered the *Bristol Approach* to cancer care, for people with cancer and those close to them. The Bristol Approach works hand in hand with medical treatment, providing a unique combination of physical, emotional and spiritual support, using complementary therapies and self-help techniques, including practical advice on nutrition. People can access the Bristol Approach through residential courses run by experienced teams of doctors, nurses and complementary therapists.

British Heart Foundation
14 Fitzhardinge Street, London W1H 6DH
Tel: 020 7935 0185
Email: bhfnurses@bhf.org.uk
Website: www.bhf.org.uk

Every 2 minutes, heart and circulatory disease kills one person in the UK. It can strike anyone at any time. Voluntary donations have helped the British Heart Foundation make tremendous advances in the diagnosis, treatment and prevention of heart and circulatory disease. However, it remains our biggest killer.

CancerBACUP
3 Bath Place, Rivington Street, London EC2A 3JR
United Kingdom
Tel: 020 7696 9003
Fax: 020 7696 9002
Cancer information helpline (UK only): 0808 800 1234 (lines staffed by cancer specialist nurses, 9 am to 8 pm, Monday to Friday)
Email: info@cancerbacup.org
Website: www.cancerbacup.org

CancerBACUP offers a free cancer information service staffed by qualified and experienced cancer nurses, and publications on all aspects of cancer written specifically for patients and their families (available in full on the website) and a growing number of CancerBACUP local centres in hospitals staffed by specialist cancer nurses. The nurses are supported by around 200 cancer specialists to help them provide the highest quality information. The database holds a comprehensive list of resources, organisations and support groups for cancer patients. CancerBACUP supports health professionals with information on controversial and difficult cancer topics written specifically for doctors and with the most comprehensive listing of UK cancer treatment guidelines.

CancerHelp UK
Website: www.cancerhelp.org.uk
CancerHelp UK can only give information on the internet

CancerHelp UK is a free information service (provided by Cancer Research UK) about cancer and cancer care for people with cancer and their families. They believe that information about cancer should be freely available to all and written in a way that people can easily understand.

Cancer Research UK
PO Box 123, Lincoln's Inn Fields, London WC2A 3PX
Tel (Supporter Services): 020 7121 6699
Tel (Switchboard): 020 7242 0200
Fax: 020 7269 3100
Email: supporter.services@cancer.org.uk
Website: www.cancerresearchuk.org

Cancer Research UK is dedicated to research on the causes, treatment and prevention of cancer. Their vision is to conquer cancer through world-class research, aiming to control the disease within two generations. They support the work of over 3000 scientists, doctors and nurses working across the UK. Their annual scientific spend is more than £213 million, which is raised almost entirely through public donations.

Carers National Association
20/25 Glasshouse Yard, London EC1A 4JT
Tel: 020 7490 8818
Fax: 020 7490 8824
Tel (Carersline – advice line for carers): 0345 573 369
Website: www.londonhealth.co.uk/carersnationalassociation.asp

The Carers National Association is the national voice of carers in the UK. Their work involves:

- raising awareness at all levels of government and society of the needs of carers and ensuring action is taken to support them
- helping carers become more aware of their own role and status in the community
- providing information, advice and support to carers, enabling them to make their own choices about providing care
- cooperation with primary healthcare teams, helping them to recognise and support carers in their surgeries
- believing that carers who want to continue in paid work should be encouraged to do so; they offer companies advice and training on developing carer-friendly policies
- pressing for guaranteed respite breaks for carers, at times that are right for the carer and the person they care for.

The Compassionate Friends
53 North Street, Bristol BS3 1EN
Tel: 08451 203 785
Fax: 08451 203 786
Helpline: 08451 232 304 (10 am to 4 pm, 6:30 pm to 10:30 pm, open every day of the year)
Email: info@tcf.org.uk
Website: www.tcf.org.uk

The Compassionate Friends is an organisation of bereaved parents and their families offering understanding, support and encouragement to others after the death of a child or children. They also offer support, advice and information to other relatives, friends and professionals who are helping the family. The helpline is answered by a bereaved parent who is there to listen when you need someone to talk to. They can also put you in touch with your nearest local contact and provide you with information about their services. The helpline also offers support and information to those supporting bereaved families.

Cruse Bereavement Care
Cruse House, 126 Sheen Road, Richmond, Surrey TW9 1UR
Tel: 020 8939 9530
National helpline: 08701 671 677
Email: info@crusebereavementcare.org.uk
Website: www.crusebereavementcare.org.uk

Cruse is a charity working to help anyone who has been bereaved. Cruse has 178 branches staffed by 6500 volunteers. Cruse works to increase awareness and understanding of the needs of bereaved people in the community. Cruse provides a range of services including bereavement support, counselling, groups and a national helpline.

Hospice Information Service
Based at two sites:
Help the Hospices, Hospice House, 34–44 Britannia Street, London WC1X 9JG
and
St Christopher's Hospice, 51–59 Lawrie Park Road, London SE26 6DZ
Tel: 08709 033 903 (calls charged at national rates)
Fax: 020 7278 1021
Email: info@hospiceinformation.info
Website: www.hospiceinformation.info

The Hospice Information Service provides an enquiry service, directories of UK and international hospice and palliative care services, electronic news bulletins, a quarterly magazine and listings of educational and job opportunities.

Institute for Complementary Medicine
PO Box 194, London SE16 7QZ
Tel: 020 7237 5165
Email: info@i-c-m.org.uk
Website: www.i-c-m.org.uk

The Institute for Complementary Medicine (ICM) aims to offer the public safe complementary medicine. The ICM established an interdisciplinary register – the British Register of Complementary Practitioners. Only practitioners who have proved to the Registration Panel that they are competent to practise can register. In addition, the ICM affiliates and accredits courses in complementary medicine, has a website containing useful contacts, and a free online journal.

Institute of Family Therapy
24–32 Stephenson Way, London NW1 2HX
Tel: 020 7391 9150
Email: ift@psyc.bbk.ac.uk
Website: www.instituteoffamilytherapy.org.uk

The Institute of Family Therapy (IFT) specialises in working with families, individuals, couples and other relationship groups. The service is available to clients who wish to work on their relationships. The IFT have a Family Mediation Service.

Institute of Psychosexual Medicine
12 Chandos Street, Cavendish Square, London W1G 9DR
Tel/Fax: 020 7580 0631
Email: admin@ipm.org.uk ; referral: referrals@ipm.org
Website: www.ipm.org.uk

The Institute of Psychosexual Medicine (IPM) is a training organisation for doctors. Seminar training is provided for medical practitioners who come into contact with patients who present with sexual problems. The IPM can provide a list of accredited doctors who accept psychosexual referrals. Please email *referral* or send a stamped addressed envelope stating the area in which you live.

Let's Face It
72 Victoria Avenue, Westgate-on-Sea, Kent CT8 8BH
Tel: 01843 833724
Fax: 01843 835695
Email: chrisletsfaceit@aol.com
Website: www.lets-face-it.org.uk

Let's Face It is an international support network linking people with facial disfigurement, their families, friends and professionals with resources for recovery. It aims to:

- offer the hand of friendship on a one-to-one basis
- link families, friends and professionals
- assist people with facial disfigurement to share their experiences, struggles and hopes
- help them build the courage to face life again

- provide continuing education to medical, nursing and allied health professionals concerning the lifelong needs of people with facial disfigurement
- educate the public to value the person behind the face.

Macmillan Cancer Support

89 Albert Embankment, London SE1 7UQ
Switchboard: 020 7840 7840
CancerLine: 08088 082 020
Benefits Helpline: 08088 010 301
Email: cancerline@macmillan.org.uk
Website: www.macmillan.org.uk

Macmillan Cancer Support provides information, emotional support, financial assistance and other practical services to people affected by cancer, including specialist health professionals such as Macmillan nurses and doctors. Macmillan has created more than 100 care and treatment centres in hospitals and the community. Macmillan is also working with patients, carers, health and social care professionals, the NHS and the government to shape the future of cancer care.

Marie Curie Cancer Care

89 Albert Embankment, London SE1 7TP
Tel: 020 7599 7777
Email: info@mariecurie.org.uk
Website: www.mariecurie.org.uk

Cancer is the UK's biggest killer, claiming the lives of more than 150 000 people annually. Marie Curie Cancer Care is challenging the disease through cancer care and research. Every year the charity provides care to around 25 000 cancer patients and their families at home and in its hospices – entirely free of charge.

Motor Neurone Disease Association

PO Box 246, Northampton NN1 2PR
Tel: 01604 250 505
Care information: 01604 611 870
Helpline: 08457 626 262
Email: helpline@mndassociation.org
Website: www.mndassociation.org

The Motor Neurone Disease Association aims to support people living with motor neurone disease to make informed choices and to achieve a quality of life. Their services include equipment loan/financial support, a local branch network, regional support workers as well as a national helpline.

Multiple Sclerosis Society

MS National Centre, 372 Edgware Road, London NW2 6ND
Tel: 020 8438 0700
Helpline: 08088 008 000
Research and Services, general enquiries: 020 8438 0742
PA to Director of Research and Services: 020 8438 0765
Email: info@mssociety.org.uk
Website: www.mssociety.org.uk

The Multiple Sclerosis Society is dedicated to a vision of a world without multiple sclerosis (MS), funding and promoting the highest quality research into MS. They also support everyone affected by MS by providing a range of services including welfare grants, information, education and training, MS nurses and a freephone helpline.

National Association of Bereavement Services

20 Norton Folgate, London E1 6DB
Tel: 020 7247 0617
Referral helpline: 020 7247 1080
Fax: 020 7247 0617
Website: www.thegrovesurgery.co.uk/shbereav.html

The National Association of Bereavement Services is a coordinating body for bereavement and loss services and acts as a referral agency by enabling bereaved and grieving people to be in touch with their nearest and most appropriate local service. The association's aims and objectives include:

- to compile a national directory of bereavement services
- to initiate and encourage regional support groups for those involved in Bereavement Services
- to provide a forum for members of the association
- to arrange training activities for volunteers, counsellors, coordinators and other professional workers
- to undertake and facilitate debate and research on matters related to terminal illness, loss and bereavement and to disseminate the results
- to highlight gaps in provision and to press for new services to be established
- to offer advice and information and to promote awareness of matters relating to the terminally ill and their families and to bereavement.

National Institute for Health and Clinical Excellence (NICE)

MidCity Place, 71 High Holborn, London WC1V 6NA
Tel: 020 7067 5800
Fax: 020 7067 5801
Email: nice@nice.org.uk
Website: www.nice.org.uk

NICE is the independent organisation responsible for providing national guidance on the promotion of good health and the prevention and treatment of ill health.

Outsiders Trust
Dr Tuppy Owens
BCM Box Lovely, London WC1N 3XX
Tel: 07074 993527
Email: outsiders@clara.co.uk

and

Outsiders
BCM Box Outsiders, London WC1N 3XX
Tel: 020 7354 8291
Email: info@outsiders.org.uk
Website: www.outsiders.org.uk

and

Sex and Disability Helpline
Dr Tuppy Owens
BCM Box Lovely, London WC1N 3XX
Tel: 07074 993527
Email: SexAndDisabilityHelpline@gmail.com
Website: www.outsiders.org.uk

Outsiders is a nationwide, self-help community providing regular mailings and unthreatening events where people meet up and practise socialising. Members appreciate a club where they are totally accepted, and some of the most amazing relationships have been formed. Outsiders is for people who feel isolated because of social and physical disabilities. The club helps them gain confidence, make new friends and find partners. Outsiders welcomes people of all sexualities, whether they are single, divorced, separated or married, and discriminates against no one. Members appreciate a club where disability is accepted and people can relax and be themselves. The first step may be to acknowledge the person's sexuality, and offer support in asserting their right to a private life, and seeking love in a society where status normally stems from good looks and money.

Parkinson's Disease Society of the UK
215 Vauxhall Bridge Road, London SW1V 1EJ
Tel: 020 7931 8080
Fax: 020 7233 9908
Helpline: 08088 000 303 (9:30 am to 5:30 pm, Monday to Friday)
Email: enquiries@parkinsons.org.uk
Website: www.parkinsons.org.uk

The Parkinson's Disease Society is dedicated to supporting all people with Parkinson's, their families, friends and carers. For advice, information or support, call the helpline.

Relate
Herbert Gray College, Little Church Street, Rugby CV21 3AP
Tel: 08454 561 310
RelateLine: 08451 304 010 (helpline where you can get to talk for 20 minutes with a Relate counsellor, open 9:30 am to 4:30 pm, Monday to Friday)
Relate Direct: 08451 304 016 (telephone counselling service)
Email: Enquiries@relate.org.uk
Website: www.relate.org.uk

Relate is the leading national provider of relationship support for couples and families. Relate works with individual families, agencies and employers to help people manage relationship issues.

Sacred Space Foundation
Contact: Jean Sayre-Adams
Emmers Farm, Sparket, Penrith, Cumbria CA11 0NA
Tel: 017684 86868
Email: Jeannie@sacredspace.org.uk
Website: www.sacredspace.org.uk

The Sacred Space Foundation provides retreat facilities and psycho/spiritual counselling (if desired) for those who are stressed, burnt out and searching for meaning in their lives. They have two sites in the Lake District. The focus is on healthcare professionals, but they accept others if space allows.

Stroke Association
240 City Road, London EC1V 2PR
Tel: 020 7566 0300
Helpline: 08453 033 100 (9 am to 5 pm, Monday to Friday)
Email: info@stroke.org.uk
Website: www.stroke.org.uk

The Stroke Association is a charity for people of all ages affected by stroke. They provide information and support through their helpline and community support services, fund research into all aspects of stroke and campaign to raise awareness of stroke and to improve stroke services.

Terence Higgins Trust/Lighthouse
52–54 Grays Inn Road, London WC1X 8JU
Tel: 020 7831 0330
Helpline THT Direct: 08451 221 200 (10 am to 10 pm, Monday to Friday; 12 pm to 6 pm, Saturday to Sunday)
Fax: 020 7242 0121
Email: info@tht.org.uk
Website: www.tht.org.uk

The Terence Higgins Trust is the HIV (human immunodeficiency virus) and sexual health charity, providing a wide range of services to over 50 000 people a year. The charity campaigns and lobbies for greater political and public understanding of the personal, social and medical impact of HIV and sexual health.

Index

Page numbers in *italic* refer to figures or tables.